Cancer Diet for the Newly Diagnosed

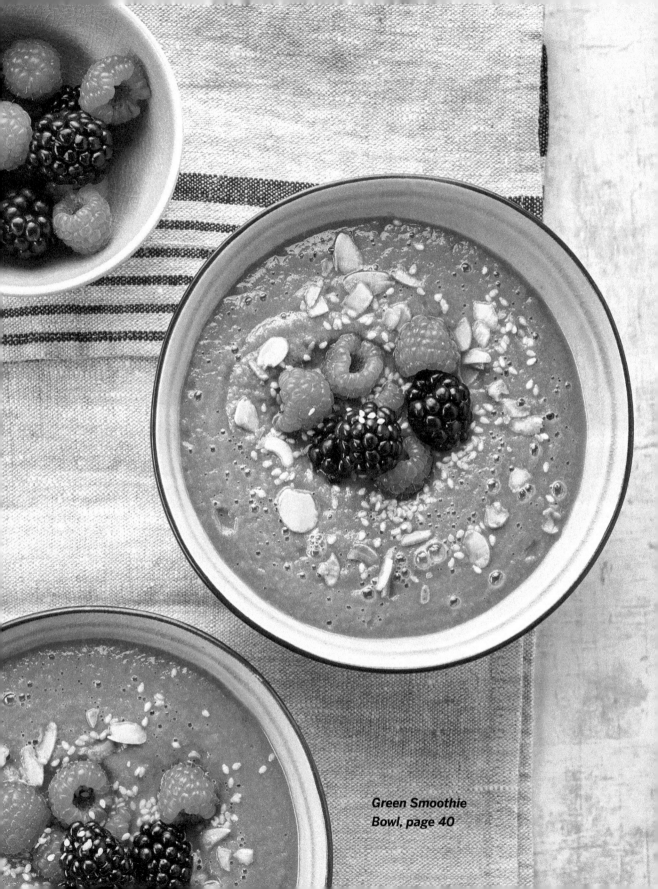

Green Smoothie Bowl, page 40

Cancer Diet
— FOR THE —
NEWLY DIAGNOSED

An Integrative Guide and Cookbook for
Treatment and Recovery

TAMAR ROTHENBERG, MS, RDN

ROCKRIDGE
PRESS

Interior and Cover Designer: Alan Carr
Art Producer: Sara Feinstein
Editor: Rebecca Markley
Production Editor: Rachel Taenzler
Production Manager: Martin Worthington

Cover photography © 2021 Hélène Dujardin. Food styling by Anna Hampton. Interior photography © Darren Muir, p. ii, 12, 30, 42, 54, 66, 80, 94, 114, 126, 138; Jennifer Davick, p. vi; Antonis Achilleos, p. viii; Stocksy, p. xi; Thomas J Story, p. xii, 28; Biz Jones, p. 2.

Paperback ISBN: 978-1-63878-037-3
eBook ISBN: 978-1-63878-266-7
R1

For my husband, Josh, in sickness and in health,
with lots of love and laughter . . . and soup.

Watermelon and Quinoa Salad with Feta and Mint, page 79

Contents

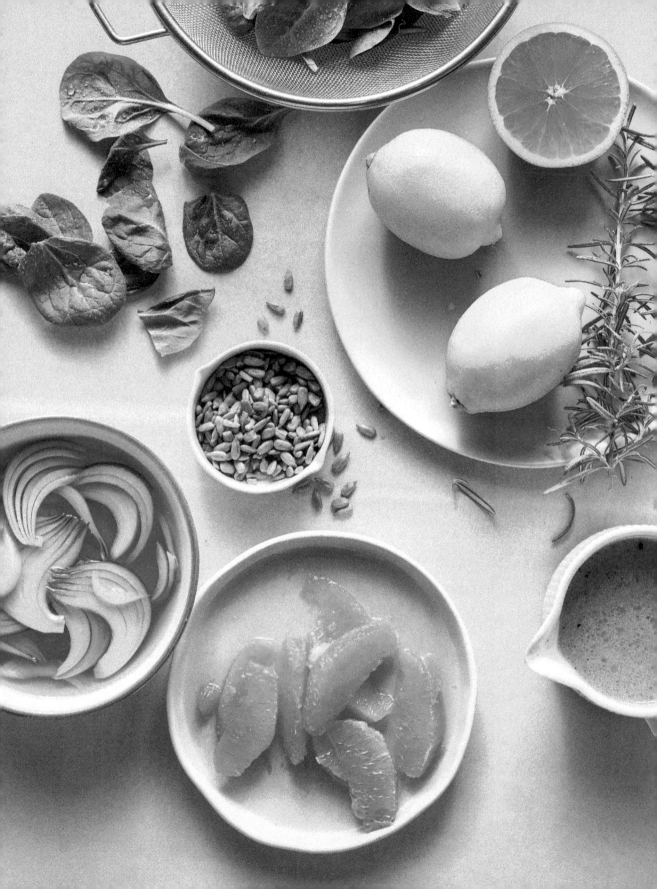

Introduction

This book is both my personal and professional mission. Having been diagnosed with breast cancer, I still remember those three life-changing words: You have cancer. You may be grappling with that right now. Surprisingly, a life-changing diagnosis can also propel you to do things you would never have accomplished otherwise. I became a registered dietitian nutritionist specializing in oncology, helping people diagnosed with cancer recover and rebuild. One result of my journey is this cookbook for the newly diagnosed.

I understand how a cancer diagnosis presents especially challenging moments for you or for someone you're caring for. From the first biopsy or scan, while waiting for results and choosing a treatment, you're on unfamiliar terrain. You may feel unsteady and powerless. There are countless decisions and appointments to make. Should you share the news with others or not? Will this be the right treatment for you?

Although you're facing difficult decisions for both you and your family, the amount of information readily available is also overwhelming. And much of the information aimed at cancer patients ranges from untrustworthy to confusing. Questions I'm often asked as a registered dietitian are: Should I go vegan or vegetarian? Must I cut out all sugar? What about eating specific foods, such as dairy, chicken, or fish?

The nutrition and lifestyle information in the following sections will help you take some control as you navigate your cancer experience. Although every cancer diagnosis and experience is different, all the treatments outlined in this book are supported by cancer organizations, oncology professionals, and cancer clinics across the United States. The science-backed recommendations have helped hundreds of thousands of cancer patients. As a dietitian, I've seen these programs in action in my own practice and in the clinical study I co-led on Cancer in the Kitchen for cancer survivors, published in 2020. Personally, I wish I had found all this vital information in one place, as it is here, when I was going through my own breast cancer experience.

Cancer Diet for the Newly Diagnosed takes an integrative approach to cancer. This means that it places the patient front and center, and that the information in this book emphasizes diet and manageable lifestyle changes during medical treatments and recovery. Evidence guides a variety of mind and body practices to support patients.

These practices include mindfulness and journaling, sustaining a support network, engaging in regular activity, avoiding environmental toxins, and sustaining good nutrition.

Work alongside your healthcare team for any dietary or physical exercise you wish to implement. Some foods and supplements may interact with a medication and even interfere with cancer treatment. Make sure to have an oncology dietitian on your team. Although this book covers some of the interactions, it cannot cover every type or other forms of nutritional support, such as enteral nutrition (tube feeding) or parenteral nutrition (IV infusion).

A new cancer diagnosis brings up many valid questions during a confusing and emotional time. There are so many unknowns. But one question that we can address is: What should I eat? My fervent hope is that this book will answer that question and relieve you of the confusion surrounding nutrition and lifestyle changes. This information will empower you to take back some of the control, to make the right dietary changes for your health, recovery, and quality of life.

**Roasted Butternut Squash
Soup with Sage, page 92**

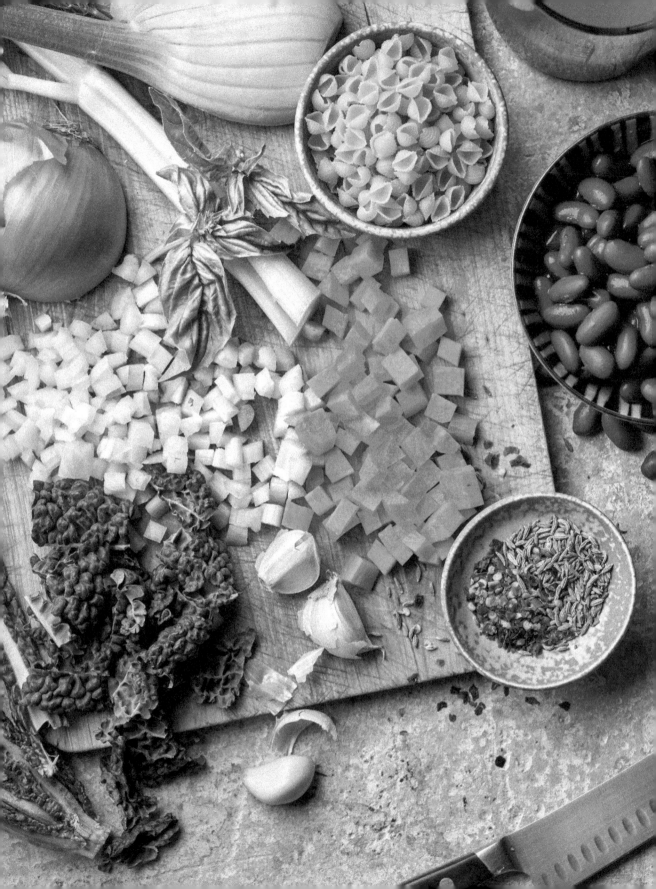

PART ONE

A Healthy Approach to Cancer Treatment

The first two chapters discuss how cancer causes changes to the body, and how these changes can be managed with food and lifestyle to help medications do their job. Using the effective strategies outlined here, you can complete treatment in the most ideal way and move forward with your life.

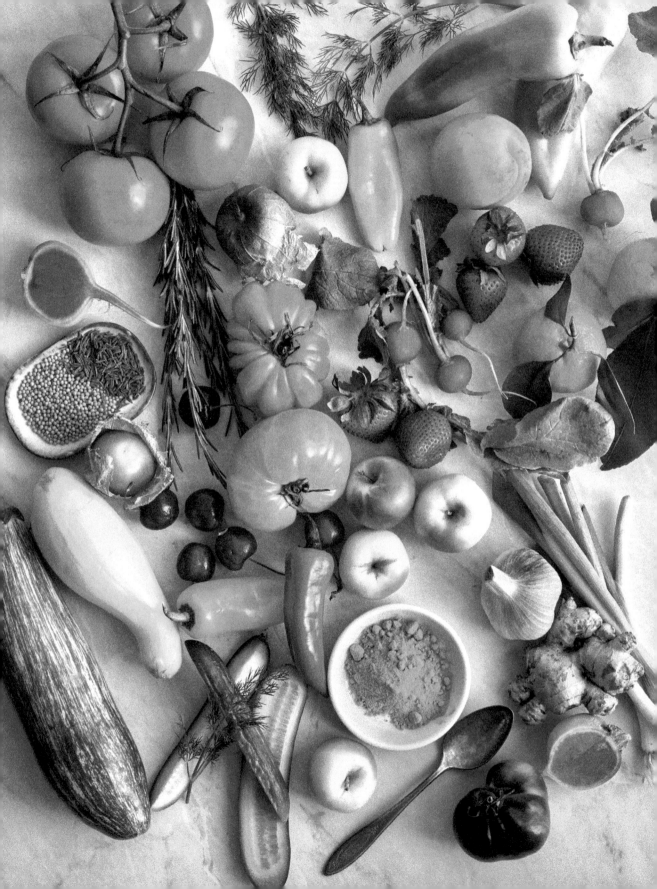

1

Starting Your Cancer Journey on the Right Foot

Think of diet and lifestyle as a supportive friend during cancer treatments. These up-to-date strategies will support you while you successfully complete treatment and help you achieve optimal recovery.

A Time for Positive Changes

Every patient with cancer is unique. No one can fully understand the physical and psychological toll a cancer diagnosis has on you and on your family and friends. One of those effects is a loss of control over your body. In an effort to help, others will be handing out a lot of well-meaning advice. But by picking up this book, you are taking on the power of making decisions for yourself that will help you on your cancer journey. It will empower you to make your own authentic lifestyle decisions, in the most efficient way possible. The best way to approach long-lasting change is by embracing small changes at the start.

This book simplifies the nutrition and lifestyle changes best suited for cancer patients. I've selected the information deemed to be most useful as you approach cancer treatments and their most common possible side effects. Every cancer is unique under the microscope, but I believe that by consulting with your healthcare team and using the guidelines, tips, and healthy recipes presented in this book, you will discover what works best for you so that you can start your treatment on the right foot.

How Cancer Affects the Body

The process of normal living cells becoming cancer cells is called carcinogenesis—the initiation of a cancer. The body tries to do its job and repair damage to the cells all the time, but when it fails to either repair or remove cells, cancer can start to grow. Cancer causes a chronic state of inflammation.

The three specific phases of cancer growth are called initiation, promotion, and progression. In the initiation phase, normal cells cannot repair themselves from damage to their DNA. Instead of damaged cells dying off, carcinogenesis moves onto promotion. Damaged cells—which should have either been repaired by DNA enzymes, or gone through programmed cell death (apoptosis)—now progress to cancer growth. The altered cells are stimulated to grow further, and move onto the third phase of progression.

In the third phase, cells grow uncontrollably, form masses (tumors), and may invade nearby tissues. Tumors measuring over 2 millimeters need a blood supply to grow, and compete with pathways normally designed for wound healing to get the nutrients they need.

When you are diagnosed, the cancer is staged, which describes how severe the cancer is, and whether it has spread or metastasized. Another factor in determining treatment is grading. Grading refers to how fast the cancer may grow. A lower number means slower growth.

Most cancers stem from solid tumors, the most diagnosed being prostate in men, breast in women, and lung overall. About 10 percent of all cancers are blood cancers, called hematologic malignancies. In these cancers, white blood cells build up in the bloodstream and marrow, interfering with the production of new blood cells and platelets. It becomes difficult for the body to fight off infections, prevent blood clots, and bring oxygen to the cells.

Carcinogenesis and its proliferation can lead to many different types of cancer—over 100 different diseases—and each type affects the body in myriad ways.

Supporting Cancer Treatment with Healthy Choices

It may seem that all decisions are now in the hands of your medical team. Yet making some small adjustments and healthy choices on your own now will put you in the best possible shape and give you the energy needed for the treatments ahead. A cancer diet is a lifestyle focusing on higher-quality foods, movement every day, rest and self-care, and managing environmental carcinogens.

DIET

A healthy cancer diet for treatment and recovery is a valuable tool in your hands. The benefits are better treatment outcomes and reduced hospital admissions and stays. After all, cancer starts with DNA damage. Numerous studies reveal that foods can repair or protect your body from DNA damage. Diet, together with movement, influences the tumor's surrounding microenvironment, making it more hostile to cancer.

The right amount and type of foods tailored to your specific condition will allow you to tolerate treatment, avoid malnutrition, and escape cancer cachexia (irreversible muscle and fat loss from hypermetabolism). Foods must be both nutritious and easily digested, because your body may respond with a faster metabolism as it fights cancer along with treatment side effects.

There is no blame or judgment for what your food choices were prior to cancer. Chapter 2 and the recipe chapters will give you the information you need now to begin following a healthy eating regimen designed to make your cancer treatment more comfortable and successful.

REGULAR ACTIVITY

Cancer researchers may not always agree on nutrition, but they all agree that physical activity can and should be done safely even during treatment. Cancer patients who exercise live longer. Exercise helps reduce cancer recurrence and releases feel-good hormones.

Any type of movement can lessen some of the disturbing symptoms that accompany diagnosis, such as depression, fatigue, anxiety, poor sleep, and ability to function. The right activities and doses do matter. A combination of three times a week moderate intensity, aerobic and/or resistance training is especially beneficial after diagnosis.

While you're in treatment, even a walk to the mailbox is a way to reduce your "tush time," says the American College of Sports Medicine. Other studies have shown that an enjoyable activity, such as gardening, improves outcomes for breast cancer.

If you're unsure or if you haven't exercised very much in the past, consult your doctor to assess any physical limitations, and ask for referrals to oncologic physical therapy before moving on to more structured cancer exercise programs. A physiatrist, or physical medicine and rehabilitation physician, can be especially helpful in recommending a plan.

REST

Sleep is the foundation of health and recovery, but up to 75 percent of people experience sleep difficulties during treatment. Coughing, pain, nausea, sleep apnea, anxiety, thoughts about the future, and hot flashes all conspire to reduce your quality of sleep. Some signals that you are in need of rest include feeling unfocused or unable to function, dizziness, and low energy. Fortunately, disturbed sleep has a remedy (aside from treating the side effects): sunshine.

Cancer cells have a circadian rhythm that is out of sync with the rest of your cells. Reset your body clock with at least 30 minutes of sunshine every day, and a minimal amount of artificial light after sundown. (When in treatment for skin cancers, ask your doctor about light boxes.) The Sleep and Circadian Research Laboratory at the University of Michigan also recommends shutting down any e-devices you use close to the eyes. Televisions at a distance don't have the same effect as a cell phone up close.

MAKING TIME FOR SELF-CARE

A cancer diagnosis brings on the anxiety-inducing challenge of juggling treatment and an already busy work or family schedule. It may feel counter-intuitive or even selfish to take time for yourself in the face of stressful and big changes, but consider self-care your prescription for decompression.

You are far from alone in experiencing a great deal of stress after receiving a cancer diagnosis. Initial stress response is highest during diagnosis and when approaching medical treatments. Then, while undergoing or recovering from cancer treatments, the initial stress response can turn into chronic stress. When the stress response is activated, the body responds with a flood of stress hormones shown to promote tumor growth.

In other words, stress—which is completely expected and normal at this time—can have negative effects when it becomes chronic, whether the effects are physical and emotional or even spiritual. Self-care, although a popular term, has a critical role in cancer care. Reducing stress supports immunity, improves the response to chemotherapy, and reduces depression associated with cancer treatment. It is not a selfish choice; taking good care of oneself has been shown to elicit positive outcomes in cancer, which benefits everyone.

Here are some ways to develop self-care as a practice:

- Think of self-care as self kindness and compassion. What would you be willing to do for a friend if they were diagnosed with cancer? Make sure you do the same for yourself.

- People want to help but may need to be told how. Don't be afraid or ashamed to ask for a school carpool or help shopping, preparing meals, or picking up prescriptions.

- Laughter is a must! Watch funny movies or have your kids (or an e-device) tell you funny jokes.

- Journaling before bed, reading books that inspire hopefulness, and taking a walk with a friend are all helpful ways to cope with a diagnosis.

One commonsense approach may include changing the timing of some medications and activities. Add light exercise, such as yoga, to your day; don't drink caffeine after morning; stop eating meat several hours before bedtime because it takes longer to digest; and set a bedtime, even if you don't fall asleep. The well-rested body will reward you with a stronger immune system.

AVOIDING ENVIRONMENTAL TOXINS

Environmental toxins interact with our genes and hormones, and weaken our immune systems. Some toxins are more obvious and include tobacco, alcohol, UV radiation, and certain viruses (such as HPV). For instance, although health benefits are touted for red wine, this does not apply to cancer patients. The ethanol in alcohol is a toxin, and cancer risk is definitely elevated by alcohol consumption during and after treatment.

Your diet may contain less-obvious toxins, which, if avoided, can mitigate more cell damage. While in treatment, it's prudent to eat organic foods because cells are rapidly dividing and absorbing more pesticides. The best seafood choices are lower in mercury (mostly smaller fish). Limit red meat to three or fewer portions per week, and eliminate processed meat (such as deli meat), as well as smoked, barbequed, and charcoal-broiled red meats and sausages. Arsenic in water sources, and in some white and brown rice, is a concern. Bottled water is monitored for arsenic levels, but check your local water supply for water quality (see Resources on page 140).

The Importance of Your Support Network

Strong social support and kindness build hope and lessen cancer pain, and studies reveal that supported patients live longer after colorectal and breast cancer diagnoses. Support helps heal the feeling of being separate from the rest of the world. A support group can give you the camaraderie you may need, validate your worries, and empower you to feel more in control over a seemingly out-of-control life change. As an alternative, many cancer patients find individual support with a therapist skilled in treating oncology patients.

You choose when and what to share with well-meaning family and friends who want to know more. Setting boundaries allows them to know you're in charge. But consider choosing to ask for support with practical matters such as meals or carpools, sorting through emotions about your diagnosis, building hope for the future, and when side effects affect your daily life.

MINDFULNESS AND YOUR CANCER EXPERIENCE

Mindfulness is about being present in the moment, observing your emotions without judgment, and finding inner peace. Mindfulness is an ancient mind-body practice with roots in Buddhist traditions. Studies show it works: Cancer patients build coping skills, find meaning, fight fatigue, and reduce the need for anxiety medications. Even sleep improves, because these practices may increase the release of melatonin.

It seems counterintuitive, but shining a light on a situation allows us to distance ourselves and notice our responses to it. We can discard what causes us to think negative thoughts, and move on to develop better coping skills and hope. Popular mindfulness practices aim to focus the mind. The following are a few known mind-body practices:

- Meditation relaxes the body and focuses on the here and now to achieve greater balance.

- Breathing exercises entail focusing on your breaths, which can help you to be more present, and clearer in your intentions and about your emotions.

- Living in the moment means finding meaning in everyday tasks, being completely present, putting down the phone, and doing one thing at a time.

- Paying attention means consciously experiencing the environment using all your senses.

Search for a mindfulness technique and the best way to access it, whether online or with a therapist, until you find a method that is right for you and that you can integrate into your daily routine.

Although it's understandable to want to remain independent, those around you may feel helpless. Most family and friends really do want to help, and you can benefit from it. You can guide them on how to offer you the type of active support that will help you cope, even if it's just making you laugh.

A diagnosis of cancer affects the entire family, and if you have young children, you may be wondering how and what to share. Always be honest, but the younger they are, the fewer details children will need. If a child needs more help, start with your child's pediatrician or the counseling staff where the parent is under medical care. Let the school know they need to be sensitive to new needs.

5 Steps to Take after Your Cancer Diagnosis

Big decisions and big changes lie ahead after a diagnosis. In addition to the broader changes outlined in this book, consider taking some specific steps to boost your physical and mental health in the months ahead.

1. **Write in a daily gratitude journal.**
   A gratitude journal develops gratitude muscles by putting positive events and people into focus. It helps negativity to fade. Try to spend 15 minutes every morning on your gratitude list.

2. **Keep a log of questions for your health team.**
   Appointments are filled with unfamiliar medical terms and new concerns. Having a list of questions with you will reduce anxiety and allow you a sense of control over your medical plan.

3. **Complete small tasks.**
   I recall staring in dismay at a chip in my bedroom dresser that I should have painted before my surgeries. The small stuff will make you sweat, so if there's anything you can do, do it now. Keep a print or online calendar for important dates and hire workers to complete small repairs in the house. Ask who can help you with small children if a doctor's appointment runs late, as they often do. Have a friend start an online community meal train for meals once treatment begins and see your dentist before treatment starts, because you may not be able to have dental work completed while in treatment.

4. **Stock your kitchen ahead of treatments.**

   Having a well-stocked kitchen can speed up food prep for nutritious meals and offer options that allow for easier digestion. See lists in chapter 2 for staples to have available.

5. **Keep a treatment and survivorship plan.**

   You may not remember the types of chemotherapy or radiation you received, so having a record of treatment in your hands will guide you throughout treatment and beyond. Cancer-specific treatment and survivorship plans, such as the ones developed by American Society of Clinical Oncology, includes the goals, side effects, lifestyle behaviors, treatments, future tests, and any other concerns that may affect your health. See the Resources section (on page 140) to download the forms.

CANCER MYTHS AND MISINFORMATION

Cancer information can range from misinformation to downright harmful information. The Alkaline Diet, celery juice for the cure, removing all sources of sugar—even fruit—and the Gerson Therapy are just a few of the unfounded and unproven diets for cancer prevention or treatment. The confusion is not surprising, given that a study found that two out of three people have no idea who to trust or believe about what causes cancer.

One in three articles on social media has harmful information, according to a study published in the *Journal of the National Cancer Institute*. This misinformation can cause great harm. Many people are led to believe that alternative treatments can cure cancer without seeking proven cancer treatments. We know that people who solely use alternative treatments instead of medical treatments have a greater risk of dying.

One recommendation is to ask your oncologist for an "information prescription" for accurate cancer information on treatments. Generally, websites run by hospitals, medical centers, government health agencies, and universities are trustworthy. Check if the article on social media has been reviewed by a medical professional.

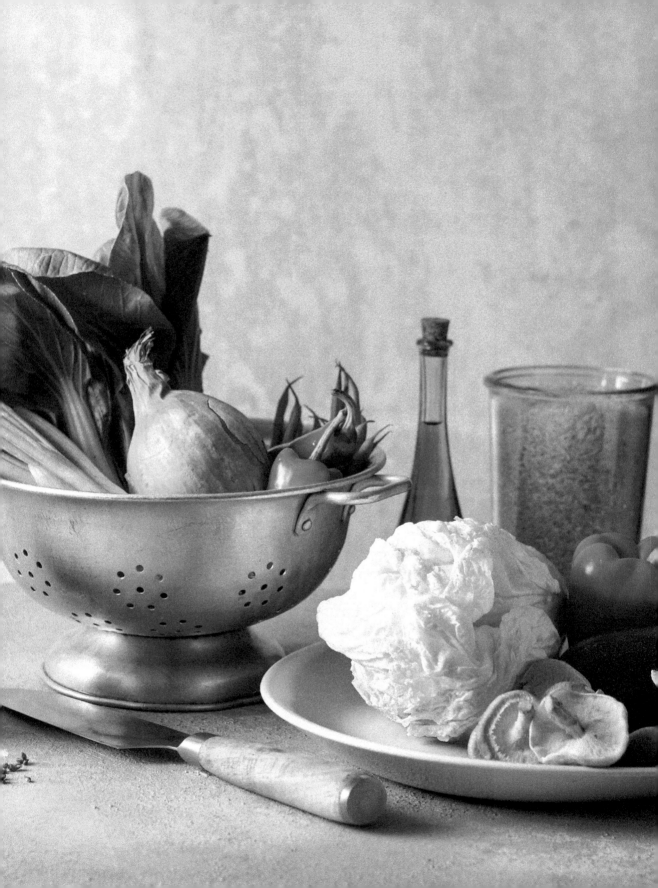

2

The Cancer Diet Kitchen

Nutritional care is critical for easing side effects and success-fully completing treatment, yet most patients report that they do not receive nutritional guidance. This chapter will explain the strong link between diet and cancer treatments. Not only is food a source of comfort, nutrition, and health, but it can serve to empower you after diagnosis.

Good Nutrition for the Newly Diagnosed

Cancer treatments must be powerful enough to destroy cancer cells. Newer treatments, such as immunotherapy, use the body's own immune system, but chemotherapy and radiation target specific areas, and may also affect nearby tissues. Dr. Susan Love, a breast cancer surgeon who was diagnosed with acute myeloid leukemia herself, calls the side effects of treatment "collateral damage."

The right mix of nutrients and calories can combat side effects and prevent treatment delays. It's important to distinguish between comfort foods and the foods necessary for our bodies to function well. By way of example, patients undergoing immunotherapy will enhance the effectiveness of the treatment by eating a lot of plant nutrients and foods that promote gut health.

FOODS TO ENJOY

Some foods have actual cancer-fighting nutrients. And other foods have properties that help minimize treatment side effects. Side effects differ in intensity in every patient, and you may still need supplements and medications, but food can work alongside them. Here are some examples: Some foods, such as citrus and pumpkin, offer antioxidants that help fight disease. Others, such as ginger and garlic, have antimicrobial effects and soothe digestion. Some foods, such as wild salmon, are anti-inflammatory. Probiotic foods, such as kefir, have antibacterial properties. Foods to combat anemia include dried apricots and dark, leafy greens such as collard greens. And the cancer-fighting nutrients found in fruits, vegetables, and whole grains will keep the immune system humming. For extra immune health, include nutritious mushrooms, along with specific foods that control cell division, such as orange-yellow squash, mango, pumpkin seeds, and chickpeas. Don't forget to add nutrient bombs—such as herbs and spices (fresh, dried, or frozen)—to strengthen the body against pathogens.

FOODS TO AVOID

Give your body a fighting chance in treatment by taking steps to avoid food illness. Certain foods not only won't help with cancer treatment, but may hinder it. Many patients think that supplements will boost their immune system, for instance, but high-dose antioxidants such as beta-carotene may actually make chemotherapy less effective and cause cancer growth. And probiotic supplements, for example, can impair your body's ability to respond to cancer immunotherapy. It's best to absorb the full array of nutrients from food rather than supplements, unless medically prescribed.

Low blood counts and gastrointestinal imbalances make it difficult to fight off infections, so they are more serious for cancer patients. Avoid undercooked eggs and meats; unpasteurized milk, yogurt, cheese, and juices; homemade kombucha and fermented foods (store-bought is usually fine); sprouts; and processed or deli meats. Also, avoid buffets, bulk bins, salad bars, and sidewalk food vendors. Don't leave cooked food out for more than two hours, including grains. Chill all foods thoroughly (below 40°F), and when in doubt about any food, throw it out.

Cancer treatments cause many eating challenges. In general, side effects such as acid reflux and even nausea can be eased by avoiding fried, greasy, and spicy foods. If you develop temporary lactose intolerance, choose nondairy options. Patients often experience cravings for sweet foods due to fatigue and steroidal medications. Be mindful that sticky and sweet foods can also lead to tooth decay, and you may not be able to schedule dental work while you're in treatment. Plus, they contain empty calories, which offer no benefits in your battle against cancer.

Alcohol is a toxin to be avoided. Sugar alcohols in food and drinks can aggravate digestive difficulties. Talk to your dietitian about fibrous foods because they will depend on treatment, such as after gastrointestinal surgery. Avoid unproven drastic diets and unfounded supplements; they can lead to nutritional deficiencies and other risks, causing significant delays in treatment.

Eating at Every Stage of Treatment

Nutritional needs change during and after treatment. It's important to consult your medical team about what to eat or avoid, and to work with a dietitian for individualized nutrition plans before, during, and after treatment.

Foods that you once thought of as unhealthy may now become necessary, such as easy-to-digest fortified white rice. Your health team may address losing weight with high-calorie foods, yet often patients are reluctant to "just eat anything." Your body may need different levels of macronutrients such as protein or carbohydrates in the short term to avoid the serious effects of malnutrition and muscle loss. Once in recovery, you'll focus on optimal nutrition and foods to reduce recurrence.

BEFORE TREATMENT

Nutrition works with medicine and is part of your treatment. You'll need nutritional stores for the surgery ahead, and there are specific recommendations for prehab. Starting a month before surgery, build up fitness with aerobic and strength exercises. You may be screened for malnutrition and require oral nutritional supplements ahead of surgery to avoid recovery complications.

Surgery requires fasting because of anesthesia. Start your nutritional prehab by increasing water intake, eating foods rich in protein to prevent losing muscle, and monitoring blood sugar as needed. Consider strategies for reducing anxiety, as well.

Preempt side effects using knowledge from your health team of what to expect from each medication and chemotherapy. To strengthen the gut in advance, increase the variety of whole grains and fruits and vegetables, and avoid fried and overly sweet foods. A low-fat diet may be protective before chemotherapy, by reversing the effects of a higher weight.

Nutritional solutions for radiation depend on the site treated and the type of side effects. Common symptoms are fatigue and mouth and GI changes. Before you start, make every bite count. Try to eat foods that are packed with nutrients, such as fruits, vegetables, and whole grains, and limit sweetened packaged foods. Healing will include maintaining calories and eating high-protein foods, especially for older adults.

DURING TREATMENT

Loss of appetite, nausea, and vomiting can accompany medical treatments. Depending on your treatment, side effects kick in within a few hours, and then resolve within a day; or begin a day later and peak at day two or three. Some side effects occur despite medications. There is also something called anticipatory response, where side effects start even before treatment begins.

Small bites and foods that ease specific side effects are helpful. Diarrhea, constipation, or sore mouth may get worse as cycles progress. It may work better to eat five to six small meals instead of three large meals. Staying hydrated is critical. Avoid fried, greasy, spicy, high-fat foods, and instead choose easy-to-digest crackers, rice, hot or cold smoothies, broths, and low-odor foods on bad days.

Even though you are very tired, don't allow time to go by without eating, because you will feel better when nourished. Eat more when side effects ease. On the other hand, fasting the day before and after chemotherapy may help prevent side effects, but always check with your doctor if you need to gain weight or recently lost weight.

In a later section, you'll find recipes suitable during treatment for taste changes (Italian-Inspired Roasted Chickpeas, page 49), nausea (Mixed Berry Yogurt Ice Pops, page 50), constipation (Everything Bagel–Seasoned Almond Flour Crackers, page 51), diarrhea (Potato Leek Celery Soup, page 82), and fatigue (Amazing Acai Breakfast Smoothie, page 32).

AFTER TREATMENT

In the weeks following treatment, you may seek to improve your health and feel good once again; it's time to rebuild and recover. You will also need solutions for any late effects from cancer treatment, such as fatigue, and to support immunity.

You may require lower-fiber foods, lactose-free foods, or low-fat foods, depending on your individual care plan. Constipation can cause pain and loss of appetite, so increase your intake of fiber-rich hot cereals or warm beverages. If you're battling diarrhea, add applesauce and rice or potatoes and reduce gas-forming foods such as beans.

Proteins, from fish and peanut butter to chia seeds, are essential if you have lost muscle mass. Exact amounts are best decided with your dietitian, especially if your kidneys are affected. Hydration, sometimes using electrolyte beverages and smoothies, light exercise, and small meals, are often key strategies for many people to build back strength after treatment.

To speed wound recovery and reduce inflammation after surgery, include fruits high in vitamin C, yogurt for zinc, and foods high in omega-3s, such as salmon.

As taste and smell aversions return to baseline, enjoy more foods and increase variety. Enhance the flavors of dishes with herbs and spices, and stroll in the farmers' market to experiment with new foods and enjoy bright colors. As you feel better, heal your gut with pre- and probiotic foods such as sauerkraut, apples, ground flaxseeds, beans, and oats.

In the year after treatment, recover by eating foods to prevent recurrence, strengthen bones, improve cognition, and protect the heart. Focus on a variety of plant foods to protect vulnerable areas that medical treatments damaged. To help heal the gut and support immunity, introduce new microbes via probiotic and cancer-protective foods such as mushrooms, garlic, beans, nuts and seeds, herbs, spices, and whole grains, along with plant proteins. Fill half your grocery cart with fruits and vegetables, and try a new recipe once a month. Find a pattern of eating—not a fad diet—that is sustainable for you throughout recovery. All cancer survivors should limit red meat, alcohol, and sugar.

In the next section, you'll find recipes for immunity (Chicken Bone Broth, page 128, or made with mushrooms instead of chicken), gut recovery (Lentil Walnut Zoodle Pasta, page 104), and simple meals for fatigue (Tuscan Chicken Skillet, page 96).

FOODS THAT HELP YOU HEAL

INGREDIENTS	CANCER-FIGHTING PROPERTIES	TARGET SYMPTOMS	HEALING RECIPES
Almonds, almond meal	Prebiotics in almonds allow immunotherapy drugs to work even better.	Fatigue Taste changes Anemia	Leafy Greens, Chickpea, and Barley Salad with Lemony Mustard Dressing (page 69) Crunchy Cabbage Edamame Slaw with Dressing (page 73) Summer Vegetable Frittata (page 41) Stovetop Steel-Cut Oats with Banana, Cherries, and Almonds (page 39)
Apples	Pectin in peel reduces insulin resistance and inflammation linked to cancer.	Fatigue Diarrhea	No-Bake Apple Date Walnut Energy Bites (page 45)
Arugula	A cruciferous vegetable, just like broccoli, with anticancer properties.	Taste changes Constipation Fatigue Swallowing Anemia	Arugula Beet Sweet Potato Quinoa Salad (page 72) Protein, Lettuce, and Tomato Sandwich (PLT) (page 74)
Beets	Beets, along with arugula, have nitrates to move oxygen through blood vessels.	Improve recovery Juice for difficulty swallowing Anemia	Carrot Tomato Beet Juice (page 122) Arugula Beet Sweet Potato Quinoa Salad (page 72)

INGREDIENTS	CANCER-FIGHTING PROPERTIES	TARGET SYMPTOMS	HEALING RECIPES
Blueberries and other berries	Anthocyanins are antioxidants in berries that protect blood vessels and brain health. High fiber.	May improve cognition after chemo Constipation Nausea Fatigue Weight Loss Taste changes	Blueberry Walnut Oatmeal (page 34) Mixed Berry Yogurt Ice Pops (page 50)
Bok choy	This is a cruciferous vegetable, just like broccoli, with anticancer properties and filled with calcium.	Fatigue Taste changes Strengthens bones affected by treatment	Tofu with Buckwheat Soba Noodles and Vegetables (page 98) Hot and Sour Soup (page 84)
Cauliflower	Indole-3-carbinol is a phytochemical only found in organosulfur plants that suppresses cancer growth—among them are breast, colon, and prostate.	Difficulty swallowing (pureed) Constipation	Vegetable Fried Cauliflower Rice (page 62) Curry-Roasted Cauliflower and Chickpea Salad (page 78) Creamy Nutmeg Cauliflower Soup (page 85) Warm Vegetable Smoothie (page 123)
Chia seeds	Protein, omega-3 fatty acids inhibit muscle loss during treatment.	Dry mouth The specific fiber in chia stops blood sugar spikes and prevents constipation	Blackberry Chia Cooler (page 125) Amazing Acai Breakfast Smoothie (page 32)

Continued >>

INGREDIENTS	CANCER-FIGHTING PROPERTIES	TARGET SYMPTOMS	HEALING RECIPES
Dark, leafy greens	Vitamin K maintains bone mass and supports brain and eye health. Prevents calcium deposits in blood vessels. If you're on blood thinners, check with your doctor so that you can consume consistent levels rather than larger amounts less frequently.	Taste changes Anemia Fatigue	"Eat Your Greens" Soup (page 93) Kale Chips (page 53) Mushroom, Kale, and Sweet Potato Brown Rice (page 65) Open-Faced Baked Eggs (page 38)
Flaxseed	Flaxseed is rich in lignans, which studies show reduce prostate cancer and breast cancer growth in newly diagnosed postmeno-pausal women. Prebiotic.	Fatigue Constipation Gut recovery	Blueberry Walnut Oatmeal (page 34) Chocolate Protein Brownies (page 48) Everything Bagel–Seasoned Almond Flour Crackers (page 51)
Green tea	Polyphenols found in green tea inhibit bladder cancer tumors, lung and prostate tumor growth. Phytochemicals block the activation of proinflammatory genes.	Nausea Vomiting Loss of appetite Feeling full too fast Mouth soreness	Lemon and Ginger Tonic (page 121)
Mushrooms	Mushrooms have antitumor compounds linked to reduced breast, ovarian and gastric cancer risk. A good plant alternative to bone broth.	Nausea Vomiting Loss of appetite Feeling full too fast	Chicken Bone Broth (made with mush-rooms, page 128)

INGREDIENTS	CANCER-FIGHTING PROPERTIES	TARGET SYMPTOMS	HEALING RECIPES
Pumpkin, sweet potato	Beta-carotene, a cancer fighter, is one of the most important phytochemicals that interact with the body.	Sore mouth Nausea Taste changes Weight loss	Pumpkin Soup (page 83) Arugula Beet Sweet Potato Quinoa Salad (page 72) Sweet Potato Avocado Toast (page 77) Mushroom, Kale, and Sweet Potato Brown Rice (page 65)
Soy	Phytochemicals in plant foods block the activation of pro-inflammatory genes; soy reduces breast cancer recurrence.	Fatigue Taste changes Weight loss (protein) Anemia	Crunchy Cabbage Edamame Slaw with Dressing (page 73) Hot and Sour Soup (page 84) Protein, Lettuce, and Tomato Sandwich (PLT) (page 74) Tofu and Veggie Skewers (page 76)
Turmeric	Anti-inflammatory spice. Studies show the active ingredient in turmeric, curcumin, may slow the progression of head and neck tumors in combination with immunotherapy drugs.	May be especially helpful for head and neck radiation side effects Nausea Taste changes	Italian-Inspired Roasted Chickpeas (page 49) Turmeric Healing Smoothie (page 117)

What to Eat When You're Experiencing . . .

Make a plan before treatment starts for days when nothing tastes good, or you're too tired to cook. Focus on protein, hydration, easy-to-digest foods, and different combinations to minimize GI distress. Don't eat your favorite dishes when experiencing side effects such as nausea, because this association will linger and ruin your favorites. Think of flavors to perk up beverages, such as mint or ginger.

NAUSEA

Nausea is a distressing yet common side effect of some types of chemotherapy and radiation to the brain, chest, stomach, and abdomen. Preempt nausea and vomiting by taking prescribed anti-nausea medications before treatment and as needed, and swallow pain medications with food. Time meals for when these medications work best. Sip cool liquids in a cup with a lid and straw to avoid odors. On treatment days or for delayed nausea, eat smaller meals with white rice, plain noodles, toast and breadsticks, bananas, ice pops, canned fruits, cool broth, ginger root or chamomile tea, bland chicken, and oatmeal. Try the Pomegranate Mint Lemonade (page 119) or Chicken Bone Broth (page 128) options. Keep your head elevated for a half hour after eating. Try hand acupressure.

FATIGUE

All patients experience fatigue, whether caused by chemotherapy, bone marrow transplants, radiation therapy, or surgery. It can also be the result of sleep disturbances, anemia, not eating enough—especially protein—dehydration, pain, and medication side effects. This type of fatigue is frustrating because it's usually not alleviated by rest.

Have easy-to-prepare, energy-conserving snacks, such as granola bars, trail mix, and dried fruit, at the ready. Prepare foods when you feel okay and freeze them for later. Eat a large breakfast when energy levels are higher, with higher-protein foods such as nut butters, eggs or tofu scrambles, and soy or dairy milk. Fruit and yogurt smoothies are an easy way to get more calories and hydration than chewing foods. Try the Mixed Berry Yogurt Ice Pops (page 50).

TROUBLE SWALLOWING

Also known as dysphagia, trouble with swallowing is often the result of head and neck radiation. Coughing, feeling that food is stuck, choking even with fluids, pain with swallowing, and mouth sores are common. Work with a speech-language pathologist to find the best food texture and other swallowing techniques. Dry foods are hardest to swallow, so use gravies and sauces on protein-rich foods or dip bread into soup.

Mashed, soft, cooked vegetables, or potatoes thinned with broth or vegetable juice, may be easier to swallow; alternate each bite of food with a sip of water. One option is Creamy Nutmeg Cauliflower Soup (page 85), but avocados, creamy peanut butter, and bananas are also nutritious choices on their own. Always eat and drink sitting up, with your head slightly forward.

ANEMIA

Chemotherapy, immunotherapy, and nutritional deficiencies can affect healthy blood cells. Pale skin, fatigue, shortness of breath, dizziness, and cold hands and feet are among the symptoms. When iron stores are low, your body needs to absorb more iron from food, so it's important to focus on iron-rich foods. But you may still need supplements. Foods that fight anemia include meat, chicken, seafood, lentils, dried fruits, and peanut butter. Don't eat iron-rich foods with calcium supplements or tea, because these impair iron absorption. Combine iron sources with foods high in vitamin C, such as Spinach Ginger Smoothie (page 116), and include folate and B_{12}, such as in the Open-Faced Baked Eggs (page 38).

TASTE CHANGES

Taste and smell changes occur with cancer treatments, but fortunately there are work-arounds: Along with good oral hygiene, specific spices and flavors will mask suddenly unpleasant flavors. For mouth sores, add olive oil and stay away from spicy food. Ask your medical team about mouth rinses.

If foods taste too sweet generally, avoid fruit and sweet juices or try diluting them and adding ice. Eat more vegetables and foods with a sour flavor, such as fermented unsweetened kefir, or add lemon juice to those foods that are too sweet.

If foods are tasting generally more bitter or metallic, avoid meat and eat more fruit, such as melon, with meals, add strong spices to those foods that are tasting acidic, or maple syrup to foods such as carrots and sweet potatoes. Use plastic or bamboo utensils, and marinate chicken, tofu, or beans in strong seasonings, as in Crunchy Cabbage Edamame Slaw with Dressing (page 73).

If foods are tasting too salty, avoid takeout foods or adding salt to your recipes; try eating more sweet foods like fruit (including tomatoes), and rinse canned foods that are now tasting too salty.

If foods are tasting blah, avoid eating frozen or canned vegetables; try eating frozen grapes, fresh crisp vegetables, and citrus fruits (unless you have mouth sores), or add pickles to a salad and vinegar-based dressings to foods with an off-flavor. Using hot (spicy) sauces may not help because they contribute heat, not flavor.

SORE MOUTH OR THROAT

Dry and inflamed mouth (mucositis) and esophagus can lead to painful mouth sores or feeling as if you have a lump in the throat (esophagitis). This can be a common side effect of some chemotherapies, radiation to the head and neck, immunotherapy, and surgery. Cold sensitivity can also affect eating. To relieve symptoms, sip liquids and use mouth rinses as directed, and avoid alcohol, citrus fruits, tomatoes, vinegar, dry and salty foods, and hot peppers.

If you don't have mouth sores, use tart foods to increase moisture in the mouth, such as frozen grapes, sugarless ice pops, and lemonade. Low-acid fruits (bananas, watermelon, and apricot nectars, among others), along with soft foods, such as creamy soups, mashed potatoes, oatmeal, tofu, custards, puddings, scrambled eggs, and yogurt, are good to eat with this condition. It often resolves after treatment. In the meantime, try the Cranberry Grape Smoothie (page 118).

UNINTENTIONAL WEIGHT LOSS

In treatment, unintentional weight loss is dangerous and can lead to delays in treatment and recovery. It's also distressing for caregivers when their loved ones lose their appetite. Fatigue, weakening immune system, losing muscle, and becoming frail are among the critical reasons to speak immediately with your doctor and dietitian about easing side effects that may cause sudden weight loss.

You may lose weight from feeling full after a few bites, appetite loss, GI distress, and pain. Some tips are to eat more when feeling better, drink only between meals, and eat smaller meals with additions such as avocado, olive oil, Greek yogurt, and dried fruit. Select high-protein drinks and nutritious broths, because liquids leave the stomach more quickly. Potato Leek Celery Soup (page 82) will help with this side effect. Eating is a part of your medical treatment. Also try light exercise to build up your appetite and help fight fatigue.

DIARRHEA

Diarrhea, or three or more additional and loose stools daily, is a side effect of many chemotherapy and other drugs, cancer types, radiation, and surgery. It can even mask severe constipation as only fluids are released. This condition can lead to appetite loss, weakness, weight loss, and dehydration. Make sure to drink slowly and often. Check with your medical team for additional medications, electrolyte beverages, pectin and banana flake powders, and taking pancreatic enzymes in the correct dosage and at the right time.

Avoid lactose in dairy, spicy and greasy foods, nuts and seeds, sugar alcohols, along with higher-fiber foods, such as raw vegetables, broccoli, corn, beans, cabbage, cauliflower, peas, onions, alcohol, and caffeine. Instead, choose canned peaches, applesauce, and bananas, pasta, white rice, mashed potatoes (potatoes contain potassium, which is needed after a loose bowel movement), oatmeal, and proteins, such as skinless chicken and turkey. Try the age-old standby, Matzo Ball Soup (page 86).

CONSTIPATION

Constipation can be caused by anti-nausea and pain drugs, radiation to the pelvis and abdomen, and calcium and iron supplements. Inform your doctor if you haven't had a bowel movement in three or more days. Anxiety, sluggish intestines from lack of movement, and low fiber can contribute to worsening constipation. Try the White Bean Dip (page 133) for extra fiber. Start your morning with a warm liquid, such as soaked dried plum juice, tea, or hot lemonade, and hot high-fiber cereal, to stimulate the bowels.

Slowly increase fiber-rich foods daily (with fiber supplements as needed) such as whole grains, raw fruits, broccoli and cauliflower, corn, beans, coleslaw, and peas. You'll need to increase your water intake proportionately with the amount of fiber. Over-the-counter stool softeners or laxatives can help alleviate the symptoms of constipation, along with medications, diet, scheduled meals, and drinking more water.

You may not get any or only a few of these side effects, but it's best to be prepared. Here's how to stock your kitchen for easy access to high-quality foods.

Kitchen Staples

While in treatment, fatigue and doctor appointments make shopping a chore. With that in mind, many of the recipes in this book use kitchen staples you can find in any local grocery store. Relying on convenience items such as canned or frozen vegetables and grains, healthy fats, and organic produce will offer the high-quality nutrition you need right now, even if they may be less budget-friendly.

Divide your kitchen into quarters to make shopping and cooking easier: pantry, counter, refrigerator, and freezer:

- The pantry can hold canned beans, vegetables, fruits, tuna and salmon, as well as quick-cooking whole grains, nuts, seeds, nut butters, plant-based milks, broths, oils, vinegars, spices, herbs, and condiments.

- The counter is for avocados, bananas, melons, and in storage, squash, sweet potatoes, and ginger root.

- Stock your refrigerator with eggs, unsweetened plain or Greek yogurt, milk or soy milk for drinks with added protein, almond milk for cooking, and flavor boosts such as capers.

- In the freezer, keep frozen herbs, grains, bagged vegetables, fruit ice pops, and smoothie packs.

Essential Kitchen Equipment

The recipes in this book do not require any fancy equipment. But key appliances, cookware, and utensils will make cooking time more efficient and conserve your energy. Keep food safety in mind: Use separate, **different colored cutting boards** for meat and produce, and an **all-purpose thermometer**. If your nails are affected by chemotherapy, preserve them using food-grade gloves. For cutting boards, be aware that wooden and bamboo boards absorb more bacteria and should be replaced more often than plastic.

Consider using "green" nonstick cooking ware such as **ceramic pans**, fewer plastic containers—never in the microwave—and Tetra Paks or pouches instead of cans to cut down on toxins. The three basic pans you need are a **stockpot** for broths, a **saucepan with cover** for grains, and a **skillet** for tofu or omelets. In the oven, choose a **large or half-sized sheet pan** for roasting vegetables, kale chips, or chickpeas.

Essential equipment will have multiple uses. A **chef's knife** is wide and long, and can be used for nearly all chopping. For flavor boosts, a **zester** can grate ginger and turmeric root or citrus zest. Use your **vegetable peeler** for ribbon-like vegetables to add nutrients to pasta sauces. Use a **salad spinner** to rinse and dry herbs, canned foods, and berries. A slow cooker and rice cooker are optional, but useful for setting and forgetting.

An **immersion blender** saves time and effort by using it directly in the pan to puree foods; and a **blender or food processor** will be used often for smoothies. A vacuum sealer with BPA-free plastic bags makes freezing leftovers easy, without freezer burn.

The Recipes in This Book

The recipes in this book are designed to nourish cancer patients and, at the same time, alleviate many symptoms associated with treatment. The recipes range from larger meals for the whole family to smaller snacks for when you may not have as much of an appetite.

The recipe introductions contain valuable information, such as how the ingredients address a side effect. For more guidance, refer to the chart earlier in this chapter on how the ingredient is cancer-protective and also targets symptoms. Every recipe has a label indicating which symptom it can treat. For example, the Peanut Butter and Banana Toast with Hemp Seeds (page 47) is a high-energy snack that also relieves constipation.

Choose from recipes labeled as just one-pot or -pan, made in 30 minutes or less, or using 5 or fewer ingredients (not including freebies such as water, salt and pepper, and oil). Other recipes are batch-cooking all-stars, best suited for cooking once and eating twice or more.

My hope is that with these recipes you'll feel empowered to make the best food choices during treatment and recovery. When you know what to cook and eat, it relieves decision fatigue. Throughout your cancer experience, the goal is for you to enjoy both your time cooking and eating.

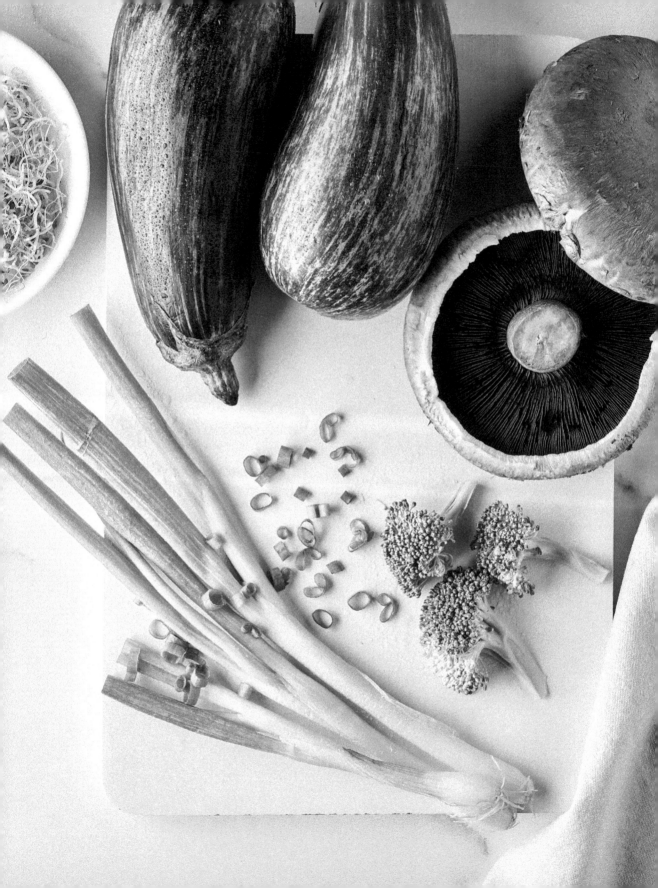

PART TWO

Healing Recipes

The following chapters feature recipes to help feed you through cancer treatment and recovery. The nutrient-filled recipes are tested for flavor, ease of use, and symptom relief. Food should be a source of comfort during this time and also help you heal.

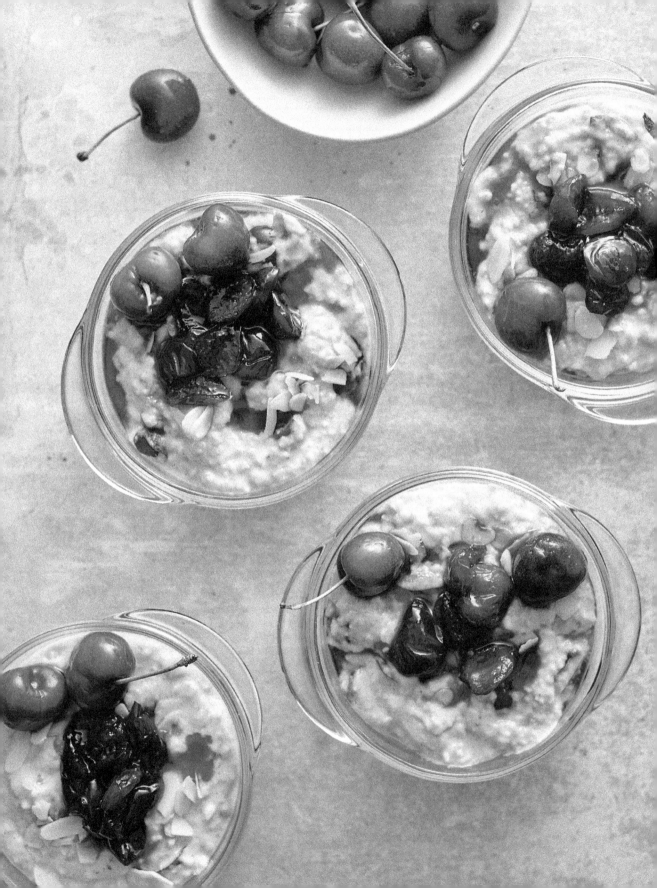

3

Breakfast

Amazing Acai Breakfast Smoothie

SERVES 2

PREP TIME: 5 minutes

GI (constipation), Mouth Soreness (no open sores), Taste Changes

Nutrition-packed chia seeds are especially beneficial after surgery, offering much-needed omega-3 fats, protein, and fiber to counter constipation from pain medications. Acai berry puree contains the anticancer antioxidant anthocyanin and more omega-3 fats, which all help to lessen inflammation. Acai berry is also tart, which helps to stimulate saliva for a dry mouth. Once mixed, chia seeds tend to clump together, so blend, let sit, and blend again.

2 (3.5-ounce) packets
  frozen acai puree
1 cup almond milk
1 frozen banana
2 tablespoons almond butter
2 tablespoons chia seeds

1 cup mixed frozen or fresh
  berries, such as blueberries,
  raspberries, strawberries,
  or blackberries, optional
Ice, for thickness, optional

1. In a blender bowl, combine the frozen acai, almond milk, and banana, and blend on high until smooth. Add the almond butter, chia seeds, and berries (if using), and blend for another 30 seconds. The mixture will thicken. Let it sit for a few minutes, and blend again.

2. Add ice and blend if you want a thicker smoothie, or add more almond milk for a thinner smoothie. Pour the mixture into glasses, and enjoy.

PREP AHEAD: If this smoothie is for one person, you can freeze half of it for another day or use an ice tray to freeze in cubes, and add as needed to drinks.

PER SERVING: Calories: 304; Total fat: 19g; Sodium: 77mg;
Carbohydrates: 28g; Fiber: 10g; Protein: 8g

Pumpkin Overnight Oats

SERVES 2

PREP AND RESTING TIME: 5 minutes and 15 minutes, plus overnight to chill

GI (constipation), Nausea (mild), Weight Loss

How about pumpkin pie in a jar for breakfast? Overnight oats solve the problem of making breakfast in the morning. Customize this dish as needed: For weight gain, add full-fat milk and yogurt. For lactose intolerance, switch up the yogurt for a plant-based option. Feel free to add more of the spices or different nuts, such as pecans.

2 teaspoons chia seeds

½ cup almond milk, divided

½ teaspoon ground cinnamon, divided

½ teaspoon ground nutmeg, divided

2 tablespoons maple syrup, divided

½ cup rolled oats, gluten-free if needed, divided

½ cup pumpkin puree, divided

¼ cup plain 2% Greek yogurt, divided

¼ cup chopped walnuts, divided

1. Soften the chia seeds by putting 1 teaspoon in each jar, along with 2 tablespoons of milk in each jar.

2. Next, add ¼ teaspoon of cinnamon, ¼ teaspoon of nutmeg, and 1 tablespoon of maple syrup to each jar. Stir well. Let sit 15 minutes and stir again, so the chia doesn't clump.

3. Divide the oats and remaining milk evenly between the two jars. The oats should be saturated but not completely submerged.

4. Layer ¼ cup of the pumpkin puree, 2 tablespoons of Greek yogurt, and 2 tablespoons of walnuts on top of the oats in each jar.

5. Place the lids on the jars and chill overnight.

SUBSTITUTION: Feel free to use dairy-free yogurt, such as oat, soy, or coconut yogurt.

PER SERVING (1 JAR): Calories: 277; Total fat: 13g; Sodium: 47mg; Carbohydrates: 35g; Fiber: 7g; Protein: 8g

Blueberry Walnut Oatmeal

SERVES 2

PREP TIME: 5 minutes · **COOK TIME:** 10 to 20 minutes

GI (constipation), Nausea, Taste Changes

How do you make food enjoyable if you lose your sense of taste and smell? Add extra texture. In this soothing breakfast, the creaminess of oatmeal contrasts with a burst of fresh blueberries and the crunch of walnuts. Flaxseed adds healthy fats, fiber, and protein, and act as a laxative. Flaxseed is the food richest in lignans, which studies show reduced prostate cancer and breast cancer growth in some cases.

1 cup old-fashioned rolled oats, gluten-free if needed

2½ cups almond milk, divided

2 tablespoons ground flaxseed

¼ teaspoon ground cinnamon

1 cup fresh blueberries

4 tablespoons chopped walnuts

1 teaspoon maple syrup, optional

1. In a small pan, cook the oatmeal according to package instructions, using 2 cups of the almond milk. It should take 10 to 20 minutes, depending on the thickness you desire.

2. Place the oatmeal in a serving bowl. Pour the remaining ½ cup of almond milk over the oatmeal, and sprinkle in the flaxseed and cinnamon. Top with blueberries and walnuts. Add maple syrup, if desired.

PREP AHEAD: Have a doctor's appointment? Store this oatmeal in mason jars, with berries as the top layer, to grab on the go. Store any extra flaxseed in the freezer.

PER SERVING (1 CUP): Calories: 434; Total fat: 18g; Sodium: 99mg; Carbohydrates: 59g; Fiber: 11g; Protein: 13g

Baked Pears with Greek Yogurt

SERVES 2

PREP AND COOLING TIME: 5 minutes and 5 minutes · **COOK TIME:** 25 minutes

GI (constipation), Swallowing (includes mouth
and throat soreness), Taste Changes

Pears have among the highest amount of fiber of any fruit and, together with flaxseed, are a delicious way to conquer constipation. The recipe is designed to address taste changes by offering layers of texture and flavor—from the warm, cooked pears to crunchy walnuts, and the sweetness of date syrup. Plus, this breakfast looks like restaurant quality on the plate. My appetite during treatment was either overwhelming or absent. It can help to try savoring the way foods appear.

2 Bosc pears
½ teaspoon ground cinnamon
¼ cup crushed walnuts

2 tablespoons date or maple syrup
1 cup plain 2% Greek yogurt,
    or dairy-free option

1. Preheat the oven to 350°F, and line a baking sheet with parchment paper.

2. Cut the pears in half, discard the cores, then use a tablespoon to scoop a circle out of the center of each pear half. Place the pears, circle-side up, on the baking sheet. Sprinkle the cinnamon over each pear half. Divide the walnuts among the four halves. Drizzle the syrup evenly over each half.

3. Cook the pears for 25 minutes. Take them out of the oven and let them cool for 5 minutes. Top each pear half with ¼ cup of the Greek yogurt, and serve.

FLAVOR BOOST: Add other spices, such as ½ teaspoon of nutmeg or ginger powder, for flavor variety. Add extra cinnamon and lessen the syrup if it tastes too sweet.

PER SERVING: Calories: 311; Total fat: 12g; Sodium: 90mg;
Carbohydrates: 47g; Fiber: 6g; Protein: 9g

Tofu Breakfast Scramble

SERVES 4

PREP TIME: 10 minutes • **COOK TIME:** 10 minutes

Fatigue, Taste Changes

Tofu soaks up any flavor you give it and, with the addition of turmeric and cumin, wakes up tired taste buds. Higher-protein breakfasts set you off on the right foot, and can accelerate healing. Help protect your bones by choosing calcium sulfate-set tofu for extra calcium.

1 (14-ounce package) extra-firm tofu
2 teaspoons ground cumin
2 teaspoons turmeric
1 teaspoon freshly ground
 black pepper
Kosher salt, optional
1 tablespoon extra-virgin olive oil

1 small yellow onion, chopped
4 to 5 garlic cloves, chopped
2 cups diced zucchini
2 cups sliced mushrooms
4 slices multigrain toast
Fresh fruit, optional

1. Remove the tofu from its packaging, and press it by wrapping it in paper towels and placing something heavy, such as a pot or book, on top for about 5 minutes. This allows some of the excess liquid to drain out.

2. Place the tofu in a bowl, and crumble it with your hands. Stir in the cumin, turmeric, black pepper, and pinch of salt (if using). Set aside.

3. In a skillet, heat the olive oil over medium-high heat. Add the onion and garlic, and sauté for 5 minutes. Add the zucchini and mushrooms, and sauté for 3 minutes. Add the crumbled tofu, and sauté for 2 more minutes. Serve immediately with a side of multigrain toast and/or fresh fruit (if using).

FLAVOR BOOST: Feel free to add other vegetables, such as chopped bell peppers, or even salsa for more flavor. Layer the spices, according to your tolerance.

PER SERVING (1 SLICE TOAST, ½ CUP SCRAMBLE): Calories: 227; Total fat: 11g; Sodium: 116mg; Carbohydrates: 21g; Fiber: 4g; Protein: 16g

Vegetable Cheddar Egg Muffins

SERVES 4

PREP TIME: 10 minutes • **COOK TIME:** 15 minutes

Fatigue, Taste Changes, Weight Loss

During treatment weeks, your appetite may drop as fatigue and other side effects settle in. This is the time to have small yet nutritious meals at the ready in your freezer, so you can easily reheat them in the microwave. These muffins are just that, and they are the perfect little vehicles to add vegetables. These have the added bonus of chopped peppers, which contain even more vitamin C than citrus fruits.

Cooking spray

8 eggs

½ cup grated cheddar cheese,
   or plant-based cheese

1 medium red bell pepper, chopped

½ teaspoon kosher salt, optional

½ teaspoon freshly ground
   black pepper, optional

1. Preheat the oven to 350°F. Lightly coat a 12-tin muffin pan with cooking spray or line it with muffin cups. (To avoid any metallic taste, use parchment paper muffin cups.)

2. In a large mixing bowl, beat the eggs. Then add the cheese, bell pepper, and salt and pepper (if using), and mix well. Divide the mixture evenly into the prepared muffin tins.

3. Bake the muffins until the tops are lightly golden, about 15 minutes. You may need to add 2 to 3 extra minutes of cooking time, depending on your oven.

FLAVOR BOOST: Add 2 tablespoons of sugar-free ketchup or your favorite salsa to the egg mixture before cooking for extra flavor.

PER SERVING (3 MUFFINS): Calories: 210; Total fat: 14g; Sodium: 234mg; Carbohydrates: 3g; Fiber: 1g; Protein: 16g

Open-Faced Baked Eggs

SERVES 4

PREP TIME: 15 minutes · **COOK TIME:** 40 minutes

Anemia, Fatigue, Taste Changes

This breakfast is attractive to both the eyes and the palate. To combat fatigue by absorbing even more iron, include a fruit with vitamin C—blackberries go great with it—or sip a fruit smoothie alongside your breakfast.

Cooking spray
4 slices whole-grain bread
1 tablespoon extra-virgin olive oil
½ medium yellow onion, chopped
1 cup sliced cremini mushrooms
½ cup chopped red bell pepper

4 cups baby spinach leaves
4 large eggs
½ teaspoon turmeric
Kosher salt
Freshly ground black pepper

1. Preheat the oven to 350°F, and coat a 9-by-13-inch baking pan with cooking spray.

2. While the oven preheats, toast the bread in a toaster oven until it is lightly browned. Then place the toasted bread in a single layer on the prepared pan.

3. In a large skillet, heat 1 tablespoon of olive oil over medium heat. Add the chopped onion and sauté for 3 to 4 minutes until translucent. Add the mushrooms and bell pepper and cook for 2 to 3 minutes, or until the mushrooms begin to brown. Stir in the spinach and let it wilt for 2 to 3 minutes. Spread the vegetable mixture evenly over the toast in the baking pan.

4. Crack an egg over each piece of toast. Sprinkle the turmeric over the eggs. Bake for about 30 minutes, or until the egg whites are set and fully cooked.

5. Season to taste with salt and pepper.

MAKE IT EVEN EASIER: Purchase pre-chopped onions, peppers, and mushrooms. Some nutrients may be lost, but it's more important to save time and eat frequently.

PER SERVING (¼ CUP MIXTURE, 1 EGG, AND 1 SLICE OF BREAD): Calories: 193; Total fat: 9g; Sodium: 235mg; Carbohydrates: 16g; Fiber: 4g; Protein: 12g

Stovetop Steel-Cut Oats with Banana, Cherries, and Almonds

SERVES 5

PREP AND COOL TIME: 5 minutes and 15 minutes cool time • **COOK TIME:** 20 minutes

GI (diarrhea), Nausea, Swallowing (includes mouth and throat soreness)

Naturally sweetened with banana, these steel-cut oats are full of fiber and are complemented by anti-inflammatory cherries and almonds. To save time, cook the oats ahead, and you can have this breakfast made in barely 5 minutes.

2 cups steel-cut oats
4½ cups almond or soy milk
1 large ripe banana, fresh or frozen

2 cups cherries, fresh or frozen, halved and pitted
½ cup slivered almonds, chopped

1. In a saucepan, combine the oats and milk, and bring to a boil over medium-high heat. Reduce the heat to medium-low, and simmer for 15 minutes, or until the oats are soft.

2. Remove from the heat and add the banana. Cover the pot so that the banana softens in the trapped heat. Mash or stir the softened banana into the oats until incorporated. Add the cherries and almonds, mixing to combine.

3. Cool the oats completely, then portion it into 5 screw-top glass jars, and garnish with more cherries or almonds, if desired.

PREP AHEAD: Store the finished dish in the refrigerator for up to 4 days. To serve, add 1 to 2 tablespoons of milk to the oats to thin the mixture slightly, and microwave it for 1 to 2 minutes until heated through.

SUBSTITUTION: Swap in rolled oats instead of steel-cut oats for a softer, more traditional oatmeal texture; just reduce the cooking time to 10 minutes. For a sweeter flavor, add an extra ½ banana. For swallowing symptoms, add more liquid of choice.

PER SERVING: Calories: 380; Total fat: 11g; Sodium: 150mg; Protein: 14g; Carbohydrates: 55g; Fiber: 9g

Green Smoothie Bowl

SERVES 2
PREP TIME: 15 minutes

Anemia, Swallowing (includes mouth and throat soreness), Taste Changes

This smoothie bowl is a highly nutritious breakfast embellished with fruits and nuts like a sundae! The added spinach cloaks its cancer-protective qualities in green. Spinach is filled with carotenoids, usually only found in orange and yellow veggies. Thicker than a regular smoothie, it requires a spoon to enjoy. You can also add granola or toasted grains for a twist.

3 cups packed baby spinach leaves
1 Granny Smith apple, cored
1 small ripe banana
½ ripe avocado
1 tablespoon maple syrup

½ cup mixed berries
¼ cup roasted slivered
   almonds, optional
1 teaspoon sesame seeds

1. In the bowl of a blender, combine the spinach, apple, banana, avocado, and maple syrup, and blend until smooth. The mixture should be thick.

2. Divide the mixture between two bowls. Top with the berries, almonds (if using), and sesame seeds, and serve.

SUBSTITUTION: Add ½ cup silken tofu to this recipe for extra protein. Pitted dates are a great natural alternative to the maple syrup, if you prefer. Omit seeds and nuts after a gastrectomy procedure or intestinal surgery.

PER SERVING (INCLUDING ALMONDS): Calories: 280; Total fat: 14g; Sodium: 40mg; Carbohydrates: 38g; Protein: 6g

ONE-POT

Summer Vegetable Frittata

SERVES 4

PREP AND RESTING TIME: 10 minutes and 10 minutes · **COOK TIME:** 50 minutes

Taste Changes, Weight Loss

A classic frittata is made in a skillet and needs to be flipped halfway through, which can be challenging. This simple yet delicious frittata is made entirely in the oven. The vegetables are first roasted in the dish, the eggs poured over, and the dish placed back in the oven to cook through. Eggs are a quality protein source and cancer patients require more protein as a healing nutrient during treatment.

2 tablespoons extra-virgin olive oil
1 small red onion, thinly sliced
1 small zucchini, thinly sliced
1 (5-ounce) can artichoke hearts,
   drained and quartered

1 cup frozen corn, thawed
½ cup crumbled feta
1 teaspoon dried oregano
½ teaspoon kosher salt
10 large eggs, beaten

1. Preheat the oven to 375°F.

2. Coat the bottom of an 8-by-8-inch casserole dish with the oil. Arrange the onion and zucchini in an even layer in the dish. Transfer the dish to the oven. Roast until the vegetables begin to caramelize, 5 to 7 minutes.

3. Add the artichoke hearts, corn, cheese, oregano, and salt. Gently pour the beaten eggs on top. Return the dish to the oven. Bake until the eggs are firm but still jiggle a little when the dish is shaken, 25 to 35 minutes. Remove from the oven, let rest for 10 minutes, and serve.

SUBSTITUTION: You can use any vegetables you'd like in this recipe, and change it up seasonally. Try mushrooms and winter squash in the winter or asparagus and peas in the spring. Store, covered, in the refrigerator for up to 5 days, but don't freeze.

PER SERVING: Calories: 341; Total fat: 24g; Sodium: 643mg; Carbohydrates: 15g; Fiber: 4g; Protein: 21g

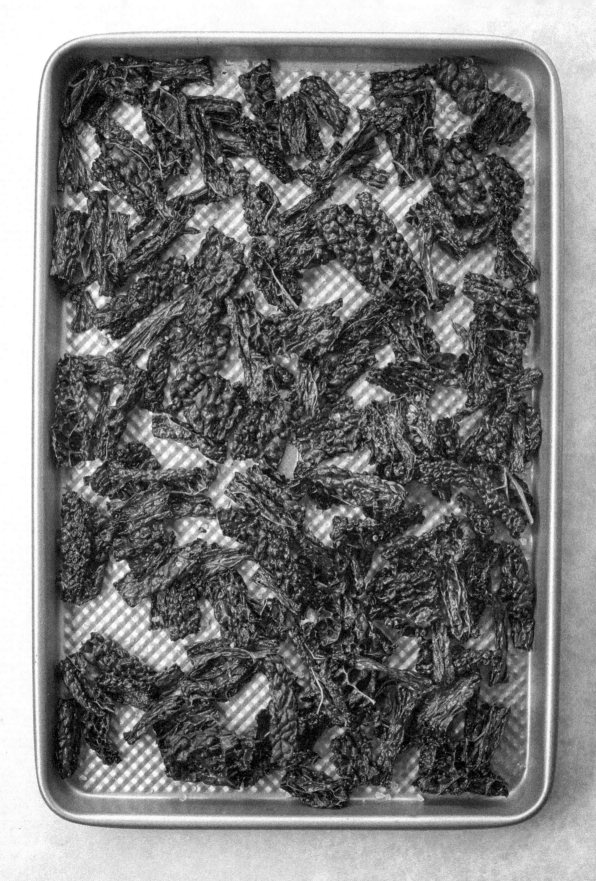

4

Snacks

Oatmeal Banana Chocolate Chip Cookies

MAKES 16 TO 18 COOKIES

PREP AND COOLING TIME: 10 minutes and 5 minutes · **COOK TIME:** 12 minutes

Fatigue, Nausea, Weight Loss

Cookies all the time? Yes, please. You probably have these ingredients in your pantry, and you can customize the nut butter to your preference. You need to pack nutrition into every bite during cancer treatments, so let's talk about the hierarchy of oats. The thinner the oats are cut, the less fiber and nutrition they provide, but the quicker they are to make. Old-fashioned oats (also called rolled oats) land in the middle of the level of processing between steel-cut and instant. These vegan cookies are easy for a caregiver to prep and freeze.

2 ripe bananas

1½ cups old-fashioned oats

⅓ cup peanut butter

¼ cup semisweet chocolate chips

1. Preheat the oven to 350°F. Line a baking sheet with parchment paper and set aside.

2. In a large mixing bowl, mash the bananas, then add the oats and peanut butter. Mix well. Fold in the chocolate chips. Drop spoon-size chunks onto the baking sheet. You can also use a small ice cream scoop.

3. Bake for 10 to 12 minutes, until the cookies are slightly browned around the edges. Let the cookies cool 5 minutes on the baking sheet, then transfer them to a cooling rack or plate to cool completely. Cookies can be frozen and reheated over low heat in the oven for 2 to 3 minutes.

FLAVOR BOOST: If the chocolate chips are too sweet, use a darker chocolate labeled 70% or higher or cut the chocolate and just add 1 teaspoon cinnamon.

PER SERVING (1 COOKIE): Calories: 99; Total fat: 4g; Sodium: 23mg; Carbohydrates: 13g; Fiber: 2g; Protein: 3g

No-Bake Apple Date Walnut Energy Bites

MAKES 12 BALLS

PREP TIME: 10 minutes

Anemia, Fatigue, GI (constipation)

If you're facing appetite loss, these no-bake energy bites are small enough to appeal, but also offer layers of fiber with iron-rich oatmeal and walnuts—plus, there's no need for added sugar because the sweetness of the apples and dates does the trick. Dates also serve as a natural way to help with constipation.

½ cup pitted Medjool dates

¼ cup walnuts

1 cup dried apples (chewy, not freeze-dried)

½ cup old-fashioned oats

1 teaspoon cinnamon, optional

1. In the bowl of a blender or food processor, combine the dates, walnuts, apples, uncooked oats, and cinnamon (if using), and blend until a thick paste is formed. You may have to press the mixture a few times with a spatula during this process.

2. Use a small spoon or a tablespoon to roll the mixture into balls. These are ready to eat immediately. Store the extra portions in glass containers or reusable silicone bags in the refrigerator for 1 week or the freezer for up to 2 months.

PREP AHEAD: These bites can be made in larger batches and frozen. To eat, thaw but don't heat.

PER SERVING (1 BALL): Calories: 67; Total fat: 2g; Sodium: 6mg; Carbohydrates: 12g; Fiber: 2g; Protein: 1g

Chocolate Date Truffles Rolled in Pistachios

MAKES 10 TRUFFLES
PREP TIME: 20 minutes, plus 1 hour to chill

Fatigue, GI (constipation), Weight Loss

Have these truffles on hand when you need a snack to help with sweet cravings or slow-moving digestion. Medications can wreak havoc with your appetite, but this combination of nuts, dates, and cacao in a pretty truffle shape is appealing and satisfying. Dates are sweet, but also more filling because of their fiber. Cacao powder is filled with antioxidants.

½ cup roasted pistachio pieces
¼ teaspoon kosher salt, divided
15 whole Medjool dates, pitted

4 tablespoons unsweetened cacao powder
3 to 4 tablespoons water (optional)

1. In a food processor, combine the pistachios and ⅛ teaspoon of the salt. Use the pulse mode on the food processor with on/off pulses until the nuts are finely chopped. Transfer to a shallow dish and set aside.

2. In the food processor, mix the dates, cacao powder and the other ⅛ teaspoon of salt. Process until the mixture forms a thick paste. You can add 3 to 4 tablespoons of water, if needed.

3. Use a teaspoon to scoop the dough for each truffle. Shape the dough into a ball, and roll each in the pistachios to coat them.

4. Cover and chill for a minimum of 1 hour before serving. Store the truffles in an airtight container in the refrigerator for up to 2 weeks.

FLAVOR BOOST: Feel free to add other spices, such as ½ teaspoon cinnamon or even a dash of chili powder.

PER SERVING (2 TRUFFLES): Calories: 278; Total fat: 6g; Sodium: 54mg; Carbohydrates: 60g; Fiber: 7g; Protein: 5g

Peanut Butter and Banana Toast with Hemp Seeds

2 SERVINGS

PREP TIME: 5 minutes · **COOK TIME:** 3 minutes

Fatigue, Nausea, Weight Loss

This toast calls for protein-packed peanut butter, naturally sweet bananas or berries, and hemp seeds for crunch and more protein. If you're taking anticoagulant medications, check with your doctor about consuming hemp seeds because they can interact. Cold snacks cut down on aromas, and are a good choice if you have nausea.

2 slices whole-grain bread

2 tablespoons peanut butter

1 banana, sliced, or ½ cup fresh berries of choice

2 teaspoons hemp seeds

Toast the bread and spread 1 tablespoon peanut butter or other nut butter on each slice. Top the bread with the sliced banana or berries, and sprinkle the hemp seeds on top.

SUBSTITUTION: Replace whole-grain bread with sprouted bread, which has begun the process of breaking down and is easier to digest.

PER SERVING (1 SLICE OF BREAD WITH HALF THE INGREDIENTS): Calories: 235; Total fat: 11g; Sodium: 169mg; Carbohydrates: 29g; Fiber: 5g; Protein: 8g

Chocolate Protein Brownies

MAKES 8 BROWNIES

PREP AND COOLING TIME: 10 minutes and 5 minutes • **COOK TIME:** 10 to 12 minutes

Nausea, Taste Changes, Weight Loss

This brownie option uses the sugar substitute stevia and bananas for just enough sweetness. When protein is paired with fructose from fruit, the combination helps steady blood sugar fluctuations. Protein powder is a valuable addition to prevent losing muscle mass with weight loss. It's usually added to smoothies, but the chocolate version can work well in desserts. Choose whey for protein powder; it is the most nutritious option for a dairy protein replacement.

Cooking spray
2 ripe bananas
½ teaspoon baking powder
½ teaspoon baking soda
1 teaspoon vanilla extract

2 teaspoons stevia
6 tablespoons ground flaxseed
2 scoops chocolate protein powder
1 tablespoon unsweetened
  cocoa powder

1. Preheat the oven to 350°F, and grease an 8-by-8-inch baking sheet with cooking spray.

2. In the bowl of a blender or food processor, blend the bananas until smooth. Add the baking powder, baking soda, vanilla, and stevia, and blend, then blend in the flaxseed. Add the chocolate protein powder and unsweetened cocoa powder together and blend once more until smooth.

3. Spread the brownie batter evenly across the prepared baking sheet. Bake for 10 to 12 minutes. Allow to cool before cutting into 8 brownies.

PREP AHEAD: Brownies can be frozen for up to 3 months. Wrap separate portions in wax paper, then seal them in a freezer-safe container to keep moisture in and freezer burn out.

PER SERVING (1 BROWNIE): Calories: 101; Total fat: 3g; Sodium: 163mg; Carbohydrates: 12g; Fiber: 3g; Protein: 8g

Italian-Inspired Roasted Chickpeas

SERVES 4

PREP AND COOLING TIME: 5 minutes and 5 minutes · **COOK TIME:** 30 minutes

Anemia, GI (constipation), Taste Changes

To help fight anemia, a frequent side effect of treatment, your body needs iron and a support system for your blood supply. The folate in chickpeas provides the support for iron and, unlike other starchy snacks, chickpeas are among the least-inflammatory foods. For even more inflammation-fighting effects, add the anti-inflammatory spice turmeric.

Cooking spray

1 (15-ounce) can chickpeas, rinsed and drained

1 tablespoon extra-virgin olive oil

1 teaspoon kosher salt

2 tablespoons dried basil

2 tablespoons dried oregano

1 tablespoon dried parsley

1 tablespoon dried thyme

1 teaspoon garlic powder

1. Preheat the oven to 400°F. Prepare a baking sheet by lightly coating it with cooking spray or lining it with parchment paper.

2. Pat and roll the chickpeas in a kitchen towel to dry them. Once dry, place the chickpeas in a single layer on the baking sheet, toss with olive oil and salt, and roast for 30 minutes, shaking the pan halfway through cooking.

3. Remove the pan from the oven, and toss the chickpeas with the basil, oregano, parsley, thyme, and garlic powder while still warm.

4. Let them cool on the baking sheet for 5 to 10 minutes. Eat immediately, or transfer to a jar or a storage container.

PREP AHEAD: You can store this snack for 4 to 5 days on a countertop in a glass container or keep it in your office drawer for when you need a protein boost.

PER SERVING (¼ CUP): Calories: 120; Total fat: 5g; Sodium: 413mg; Carbohydrates: 15g; Fiber: 5g; Protein: 4g

Mixed Berry Yogurt Ice Pops

MAKES 8 ICE POPS

PREP TIME: 15 minutes, plus 4 hours to freeze

Nausea, Swallowing (includes mouth and throat soreness), Taste Changes

Frozen fruit ice pops are soothing to a dry mouth, and tend to be a welcome food when someone is experiencing sudden taste changes and nausea. Berries are not appropriate if you have mouth sores, but they offer vitamin C for healing wounds and help build collagen after surgery. The benefit of making these at home is adding just the right amount and type of sweetness, and avoiding ingredients such as sugar alcohols that can aggravate digestive difficulties.

2 cups mixed berries, fresh, or frozen and thawed (see Substitution for mouth sores)

2 tablespoons maple syrup, divided
1 cup plain 2% Greek yogurt

1. In the bowl of a blender or food processor, puree the berries until smooth. Transfer the berry mixture to a medium bowl, and stir in 1 tablespoon of maple syrup.

2. In a small bowl, mix the yogurt and the other tablespoon of maple syrup until well combined. Add the yogurt and maple syrup mixture to the berry puree, and mix to combine.

3. Pour the ice-pop mixture into ice-pop molds and insert ice-pop sticks. Freeze for at least 4 hours.

SUBSTITUTION: There are many ways to customize these ice pops to taste. Use dairy-free yogurt, such as that based on coconut or oat milk, if you prefer. If they taste too sweet, omit the maple syrup. For a tarter taste, use only blackberries, but they will contain small seeds. If you have mouth sores, try grapes (2 cups, fresh or frozen) or watermelon instead of the berries.

PER SERVING (1 ICE POP): Calories: 49; Total fat: 1g; Sodium: 15mg; Carbohydrates: 9g; Fiber: 2g; Protein: 2g

Everything Bagel–Seasoned Almond Flour Crackers

MAKES 30 TO 35 CRACKERS
PREP AND COOLING TIME: 5 minutes and 5 minutes · **COOK TIME:** 22 to 25 minutes

GI (constipation), Nausea

Plain crackers are often the go-to for nausea or gastrointestinal difficulties, but after a while, the bland flavor may become unappealing. Try making crackers at home, and perfecting the recipe with seasonings you not only tolerate, but enjoy. Almond flour is grain-free and, although not fortified like white flour, does contain a high amount of magnesium. It even provides a source of prebiotics to help your gut heal.

1 cup almond flour
1 tablespoon ground flaxseed
3 tablespoons water

1 teaspoon sea salt
2 to 3 tablespoons everything
   bagel seasoning

1. Preheat the oven to 350°F, and line a baking sheet with parchment paper.

2. In a medium bowl, mix together the flour, flaxseed, water, and salt until a dough forms.

3. Place the dough on the baking sheet, and place another piece of parchment paper on top of it. Use your hands or a rolling pin to roll the dough out to about ¼-inch thickness. You will want it on the thinner side so that it will have a cracker-like texture.

4. Remove the top piece of parchment, and add the everything bagel seasoning to your taste. You can press it in a bit with your hands, or the parchment paper, before putting the pan in the oven.

5. Bake the crackers for 22 to 25 minutes. Take the crackers out of the oven when they are slightly brown around the edges, and let them cool for 5 to 7 minutes. Cut into 2-by-2-inch pieces, and enjoy. These crackers will keep in an airtight container on your counter for 5 days or in the freezer for up to 2 months.

PER SERVING (5 CRACKERS): Calories: 98; Total fat: 8g; Sodium: 291mg; Carbohydrates: 4g; Fiber: 2g; Protein: 4g

Nut Butter Shortbread

MAKES 16 COOKIE BARS

PREP AND COOLING TIME: 10 minutes and 30 minutes • **COOK TIME:** 20 minutes

Anemia, Weight Loss

Shortbread cookies are delicious, but usually contain copious amounts of butter. By using peanut butter instead, you achieve the same creaminess, increase your protein intake, and add a satisfying flavor boost. Factor in the iron provided by the walnuts, and you have a well-balanced snack perfect for any time of day.

3 tablespoons maple syrup
½ cup creamy peanut butter
1 large egg
½ teaspoon vanilla extract

¼ teaspoon baking soda
¼ cup mini chocolate chips
16 raw walnut halves

1. Preheat the oven to 350°F, and line an 8-by-8-inch pan with parchment paper.

2. In a medium mixing bowl, whisk together the maple syrup, peanut butter, egg, vanilla, and baking soda. Fold in the mini chocolate chips.

3. Press the batter into the pan with your hands. It doesn't need to reach all the way to the edges. To create cookies, score the batter with your knife to make 16 squares, but don't cut all the way through. Top with a walnut on each cookie.

4. Bake for 20 minutes. Let them cool for 30 minutes before cutting all the way through. The cookies harden as they cool.

SUBSTITUTION: Use cashew butter, crunchy peanut butter, or a chocolate-peanut butter mix (omit the chocolate chips) for a different take on this recipe. All these nut butters have just the right amount of creaminess.

PER SERVING (1 COOKIE): Calories: 101; Total fat: 7g; Sodium: 60mg; Carbohydrates: 6g; Fiber: 1g; Protein: 3g

Kale Chips

SERVES 4

PREP TIME: 10 minutes · **COOK TIME:** 20 minutes

Anemia

Kale is a powerhouse vegetable. This cancer-protective leafy green is a cruciferous veggie, in the same family as broccoli, and remarkably high in nutrients. This recipe makes delicious chips at a fraction of the price of store-bought kale chips. You know exactly what's in them, and are assured you're getting maximum nutrition. If you like it spicy, add a pinch of red pepper flakes to the kale before baking.

Cooking spray

1 large bunch kale, washed
 and thoroughly dried, stems
 removed, cut into 2-inch pieces

2 tablespoons extra-virgin olive oil

1 teaspoon sea salt

1. Preheat the oven to 275°F. Coat a large baking sheet with cooking spray.

2. In a large bowl, use your hands to mix the kale and olive oil until the kale is evenly coated. Transfer the kale to a large baking sheet, and sprinkle the sea salt over it.

3. Bake, turning the kale leaves once halfway through, until crispy, about 20 minutes.

PREP AHEAD: It's best to enjoy these kale chips within 24 hours of making them, because they lose their crunch quickly. Keep them in an airtight container at room temperature.

PER SERVING: Calories: 88; Total fat: 7g; Sodium: 605mg;
Carbohydrates: 6g; Fiber: 2g; Protein: 2g

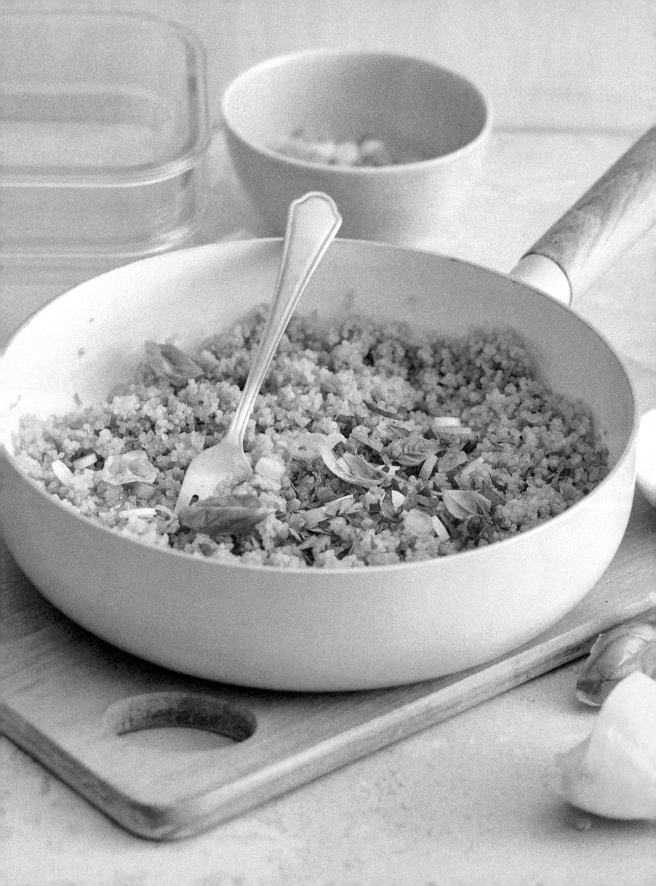

5

Vegetables and Sides

Swiss Chard and Kale with Sesame and Garlic

SERVES 2

PREP TIME: 5 minutes • **COOK TIME:** 7 minutes

Anemia, Fatigue, Taste Changes

At times, you won't want to eat a leafy green in sight. But when you do, this dish can offer you the nutrients your heart needs, such as iron, calcium, and potassium. Use pre-chopped kale to lessen your time in the kitchen. Coconut aminos may be an unfamiliar condiment for you, but they contain much less sodium than soy sauce.

1 bunch Swiss chard

1 bunch lacinato kale

2 tablespoons sesame oil

¼ cup sesame seeds

4 garlic cloves, minced

1 red bell pepper (or orange or yellow pepper), thinly sliced

1 tablespoon coconut aminos

1. Separate the stems and leaves of the Swiss chard, chop them separately, and divide into two piles, one for stems and one for leaves. Repeat with the kale.

2. In a shallow frying pan, heat the sesame oil over medium heat for 1 minute, then roast the sesame seeds until lightly toasted. Add the garlic, and sauté for 30 seconds. Remove this mixture from the pan, and set aside.

3. Put the chard and kale stems in the pan and sauté for 2 minutes over medium heat. Add the bell pepper, and sauté for 1 minute. Add the chard and kale leaves, cover, and cook for about 3 minutes, just until wilted. Season with coconut aminos, and turn off the heat. Add the sesame seed/garlic mixture, mix well, and serve.

FLAVOR BOOST: You can substitute ½ tablespoon reduced-sodium soy sauce if you do not like the flavor of coconut aminos. Add a squeeze of lemon when serving, to absorb even more iron from the leafy greens.

PER SERVING (1 CUP): Calories: 310; Total fat: 26g; Sodium: 90mg; Carbohydrates: 16g; Fiber: 7g; Protein: 9g

Brussels Sprouts with Dijon Mustard Sauce

SERVES 4

PREP TIME: 5 minutes · **COOK TIME:** 20 minutes

GI (constipation), Taste Changes

Because constipation is a frequent side effect, it's best to prevent being uncomfortable during treatment by adding fiber to your meals. Try a serving of vegetables or fruit with most meals, as tolerated. Roasting Brussels sprouts brings out their sweetness, and the addition of a mustard and apple cider vinegar dressing allows strong flavors to hit the tongue first and signal food enjoyment.

12 fresh Brussels sprouts, trimmed and halved

2 tablespoons extra-virgin olive oil, divided

1 teaspoon kosher salt, divided

1 teaspoon freshly ground black pepper, divided

1 tablespoon apple cider vinegar

2 tablespoons Dijon mustard

1. Preheat the oven to 450°F. Line a large baking sheet with parchment paper.

2. In a large bowl, toss the Brussels sprouts with 1 tablespoon of oil and ½ teaspoon each of the salt and pepper. Move the sprouts to the prepared baking sheet. Roast them for 10 minutes, then toss, and roast 10 more minutes.

3. While the sprouts cook, in a medium mixing bowl, whisk together the vinegar, the mustard, the other tablespoon of olive oil, and the remaining salt and pepper.

4. Add the roasted sprouts to the dressing, and toss them around to coat them fully. Transfer them to a platter and serve.

FLAVOR BOOST: Add a broiled chicken breast or seitan and a roasted sweet potato, or add a piece of your favorite fish and ½ cup rice to make this dish more satisfying.

PER SERVING (½ CUP BRUSSELS SPROUTS): Calories: 90; Total fat: 7g; Sodium: 391mg; Carbohydrates: 6g; Fiber: 3g; Protein: 2g

Savory Cauliflower Muffins

MAKES 12 MUFFINS
PREP TIME: 10 minutes · **COOK TIME:** 15 minutes

GI (Constipation), Taste Changes, Weight Loss

This recipe is an easy way to increase your veggie servings, but with a fun muffin twist. Feel free to spice the muffins the way you want; cauliflower is just a backdrop for the flavors you add. I encourage you to use frozen pre-riced cauliflower because it's as nutritious as whole cauliflower and is a great time-saver. Just let it defrost on the counter for a few minutes, so it's easier to mix with the eggs.

Cooking spray
3 eggs
1 onion, chopped
1 bag riced cauliflower, frozen
  and thawed, or fresh
1 teaspoon ground cumin

1 teaspoon garlic powder
1 teaspoon paprika
½ teaspoon kosher salt
½ teaspoon freshly ground
  black pepper, optional

1. Preheat the oven to 425°F, and lightly coat a 12-tin muffin pan with cooking spray or line it with muffin cups.

2. In a medium mixing bowl, beat the eggs. Then add the onion, riced cauliflower, cumin, garlic powder, paprika, salt, and pepper (if using), and mix until well combined.

3. Divide the mixture evenly into the prepared muffin tins. Bake until the tops are lightly browned, about 15 minutes. You may need to add 2 to 3 extra minutes of cooking time, depending on your oven.

4. Leftover muffins can be stored in the refrigerator for 4 days or in an airtight container in the freezer for up to 3 months.

PER SERVING (2 MUFFINS): Calories: 58; Total fat: 3g; Sodium: 148mg; Carbohydrates: 5g; Fiber: 2g; Protein: 4g

Layered Greek-Style Vegetables

SERVES 4

PREP AND REST TIME: 15 minutes and 10 minutes • **COOK TIME:** 30 to 40 minutes

GI (constipation), Swallowing (includes mouth
and throat soreness), Taste Changes

Vegetables are layered in a Dutch oven and baked, which makes this a great candidate for leftovers to warm in the microwave. Serve ladled over a thick slice of bread. Make sure to use pasteurized milk and cheeses for food safety.

¼ cup extra-virgin olive oil
1 medium white onion, thinly sliced
2 large zucchini, thinly sliced
2 cups cauliflower florets
1 fennel bulb, trimmed
  and thinly sliced
2 garlic cloves, minced

1 teaspoon kosher salt
¼ teaspoon freshly ground
  black pepper
2 cups vegetable broth
1 tablespoon chopped fresh dill
1½ teaspoons grated lemon zest
½ cup crumbled feta, optional

1. Preheat the oven to 400°F. Pour the oil into a Dutch oven. Arrange the onion in a single layer, and top, in layers, with the zucchini, cauliflower, fennel, garlic, salt, and pepper.

2. Pour the broth over the vegetables, and sprinkle with the dill and lemon zest. Put the lid on the pot, transfer it to the oven, and roast until the vegetables are tender, 30 to 40 minutes.

3. Remove from the oven, and let it rest for about 10 minutes. Sprinkle with the feta (if using) and serve. The vegetables can be stored, covered, in the refrigerator for up to 5 days or in the freezer for several months.

FLAVOR BOOST: You can easily amp up the flavor and protein in this dish by adding drained cooked beans or cooked chicken.

PER SERVING: Calories: 200; Total fat: 14g; Sodium: 1,028mg;
Carbohydrates: 17g; Fiber: 6g; Protein: 7g

Cauliflower Tabbouleh

SERVES 4

PREP AND RESTING TIME: 10 minutes and 15 minutes

Fatigue, GI (constipation), Nausea (mild), Taste Changes

This recipe is a grain-free alternative to tabbouleh, which is a traditional Middle Eastern summer dish made with cracked bulgur wheat. Patients may develop sensitivities and find grain difficult to digest at times, so cauliflower is a perfect substitution. Lemon and mint brighten this dish, and cucumbers add much-needed hydration. When taste changes make food taste bitter, lemon juice and other herbs can mask flavors and perk up taste.

3 cups riced cauliflower

1 cup coarsely chopped parsley

1 cup coarsely chopped fresh mint

2 garlic cloves, finely chopped

½ cup chopped cilantro

2 cups diced cherry tomatoes

1 cup chopped Persian cucumber

2 tablespoons freshly
squeezed lemon juice

4 tablespoons extra-virgin olive oil

Kosher salt

Freshly ground black pepper

In a medium bowl, combine the riced cauliflower, parsley, mint, garlic, cilantro, chopped tomatoes, and cucumber. Add the lemon juice and olive oil. Add salt and pepper to taste. Toss it a bit. Let the salad sit for 10 to 15 minutes before serving.

FLAVOR BOOST: Add scallions for a flavor boost.

SUBSTITUTION: For mild nausea, cooked white rice might be a better option than cauliflower; skip the olive oil and tomatoes, and add pressed ginger juice instead.

PER SERVING (½ CUP): Calories: 183; Total fat: 14g; Sodium: 85mg; Carbohydrates: 13g; Fiber: 5g; Protein: 4g

Savory Herbed Quinoa

MAKES 3½ CUPS

PREP AND REST TIME: 5 minutes and 10 minutes • **COOK TIME:** 15 minutes

Anemia, GI (Constipation), Swallowing (includes mouth and throat soreness)

Quinoa, a protein-heavy seed (often thought of as a grain), has a very mild flavor, but when prepared with savory herbs and seasoning it becomes a delicious and versatile side dish. Fresh parsley, basil, and scallions add depth of flavor to this recipe, in addition to anti-inflammatory benefits. Add more broth before serving to make it easier to chew and swallow.

1 cup quinoa, rinsed

2 cups vegetable broth

1½ tablespoons extra-virgin olive oil

Juice of ½ lemon

½ teaspoon kosher salt

½ teaspoon freshly ground black pepper

½ cup chopped fresh parsley

½ cup chopped fresh basil

2 scallions, white and green parts, chopped

1. In a saucepan, combine the quinoa and broth, and bring to a boil over high heat. Reduce the heat to medium-low, cover, and simmer for 15 to 20 minutes, or until the liquid is absorbed and the quinoa looks fluffy. Remove from the heat and let it rest, covered, for 10 minutes.

2. Transfer the cooked quinoa to a large serving bowl, and add the olive oil, lemon juice, salt, pepper, parsley, basil, and scallions. Stir to incorporate, and serve.

PREP AHEAD: Store the quinoa in an airtight container in the refrigerator for up to 5 days. Freeze quinoa for up to 2 months and thaw it in the refrigerator overnight before reheating in the microwave. You can also cook double the amount of quinoa and divide it in half. Add the herbs used in this recipe to one portion and keep the remaining quinoa plain to use in other recipes.

PER SERVING (SCANT ¾ CUP): Calories: 175; Total fat: 6g; Sodium: 321mg; Carbohydrates: 25g; Fiber: 3g; Protein: 5g

Vegetable Fried Cauliflower Rice

SERVES 4

PREP TIME: 15 minutes · **COOK TIME:** 15 minutes

Anemia, Nausea, Taste Changes

Cauliflower rice is the key to an anti-inflammatory stir-fry. Perfectly balanced with protein from nutrient-dense tofu, this satisfying and flavorful dish is packed with vegetables, herbs, and spices. In this recipe, you'll make a simple homemade version of stir-fry sauce, with less salt than that found in store-bought options.

Garlic-Herb Marinated
 Tofu (page 132)
3 tablespoons tamari
½ teaspoon honey
1 teaspoon rice vinegar
1 tablespoon coconut oil
1 carrot, sliced into thin rounds
2 garlic cloves, minced
1 tablespoon finely chopped
 fresh ginger

1 tablespoon water
1 (12-ounce) package frozen
 riced cauliflower, or one
 head cauliflower, riced
1 cup green peas, fresh or frozen
1 tablespoon sesame oil
2 large eggs, beaten
2 scallions, white and
 green parts, minced

1. Preheat the oven and marinate the tofu as directed in the recipe for Garlic-Herb Marinated Tofu (steps 1 to 3).

2. In a small bowl, whisk together the tamari, honey, and vinegar. Set it aside. Move the tofu to the oven (step 4 of the recipe for Garlic-Herb Marinated Tofu).

3. While the tofu bakes, in a large skillet, heat the coconut oil over medium heat. Add the carrot, garlic, and ginger, and cook, stirring often, for 3 to 4 minutes, or until the carrot softens and the garlic is fragrant. If the mixture is dry, add water 1 teaspoon at a time so the carrots can continue cooking.

4. Add the riced cauliflower and peas to the skillet. Stir frequently to stir-fry the cauliflower until it softens and then begins to crisp, 4 to 7 minutes.

5. Make a well in the middle of the cauliflower mixture and add the sesame oil. Heat the oil for 30 seconds, then pour the eggs on top of the oil. Stir the eggs constantly to scramble them, 2 to 3 minutes, until fully cooked. Stir the cooked eggs into the mixture. Add the tamari, honey, and vinegar mixture to the skillet, and stir to coat.

6. Remove the tofu from the oven and set it aside to cool. Serve the cauliflower rice topped with the tofu and scallions.

PREP AHEAD: Store in the refrigerator. To serve, microwave for 1 to 2 minutes or until warmed through. In an airtight container, this rice may be frozen for up to 2 months. Thaw overnight in the refrigerator before reheating.

PER SERVING: Calories: 318; Total fat: 23g; Sodium: 1,124g; Carbohydrates: 16g; Fiber: 3g; Protein: 18g

Garlicky Cannellini Beans

SERVES 4 TO 6

PREP TIME: 10 minutes • **COOK TIME:** 15 minutes

Anemia, GI (constipation), Taste Changes

Swiss chard, cannellini beans, and garlic are the hearty base for this dish. The beans have layers of nutrition needed now, with protein, fiber, magnesium for strong bones, and minerals such as iron and calcium to fight anemia. Sop up the juices with some soft whole-grain bread.

1 large bunch Swiss chard, leaves only, cut into 2-inch strips
1 (15-ounce) can cannellini beans, drained and rinsed
1 cup vegetable broth
½ small onion, chopped
¼ cup extra-virgin olive oil

2 garlic cloves, thinly sliced
1 teaspoon grated lemon zest
1 teaspoon kosher salt
½ teaspoon dried rosemary
2 tablespoons freshly squeezed lemon juice

1. Preheat the oven to 400°F.

2. In an 8-by-8-inch casserole dish, combine the Swiss chard, beans, broth, onion, oil, garlic, lemon zest, salt, and rosemary, and stir until well mixed.

3. Cover the dish, transfer to the oven, and bake until the chard has wilted and the beans are thoroughly heated, 10 to 15 minutes. Stir in the lemon juice, and serve.

PREP AHEAD: Leftovers are great eaten as a cold salad. Store, covered, in the refrigerator for up to 5 days or in the freezer for several months.

PER SERVING: Calories: 217; Total fat: 14g; Sodium: 853mg; Carbohydrates: 18g; Fiber: 6g; Protein: 8g

ONE-POT

Mushroom, Kale, and Sweet Potato Brown Rice

SERVES 4

PREP TIME: 10 minutes · **COOK TIME:** 50 minutes

GI (diarrhea), Nausea, Swallowing (includes mouth and throat soreness)

Brown rice has additional fiber to help with constipation, but you can switch to white rice if nausea is more severe. The vegetables are soft enough to enable patients with chewing difficulties to eat.

¼ cup extra-virgin olive oil

4 cups coarsely chopped kale leaves

2 leeks, white parts only, thinly sliced

1 cup sliced mushrooms

2 garlic cloves, minced

2 cups peeled (½-inch cubed) sweet potatoes

1 cup brown rice

2 cups vegetable broth

1 teaspoon kosher salt

¼ teaspoon freshly ground black pepper

¼ cup freshly squeezed lemon juice

2 tablespoons finely chopped fresh flat-leaf parsley

1. In a Dutch oven, heat the oil over high heat. Add the kale, leeks, mushrooms, and garlic, and sauté until soft, about 5 minutes. Add the sweet potatoes and rice, and sauté for about 3 minutes. Add the broth, salt, and pepper, and bring to a boil.

2. Reduce the heat to a simmer and cook, partially covered, until the rice is tender, 30 to 40 minutes. Take it off the heat, stir in the lemon juice and parsley, and serve. The rice can be stored, covered, in the refrigerator for up to 5 days or in the freezer for several months.

SUBSTITUTION: Feel free to substitute any green of choice for the kale. Swiss chard, mustard greens, or spinach all work well.

PER SERVING: Calories: 425; Total fat: 15g; Sodium: 1,045mg; Carbohydrates: 65g; Fiber: 6g; Protein: 11g

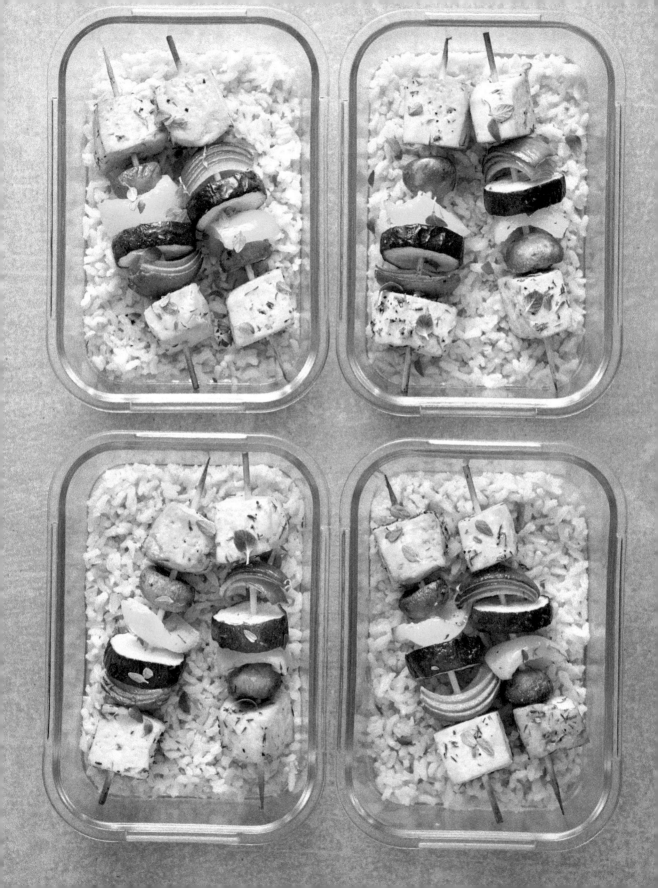

6

Salads and Handhelds

Spinach Raspberry Walnut Salad

SERVES 2

PREP TIME: 5 minutes

Anemia, Fatigue, Taste Changes

A refreshing spinach-raspberry combination adds just the right amount of tartness you need to combat off-tastes. Layers of texture, from the leafy spinach to soft feta and crunchy walnuts, add a much-needed twist when food tastes flavorless. Taste changes can hit suddenly, and it's a bit of a shock to lose the enormous comfort that food provides. It was hard for me to believe that my ability to taste would return, but it did, and with gusto.

2 pints fresh raspberries, divided

½ cup balsamic vinegar

Kosher salt

Black pepper

1 cup extra-virgin olive oil

4 cups baby spinach leaves

¼ cup crushed walnuts

2 tablespoons crumbled feta

1. In the bowl of a food processor, combine 1 pint of the raspberries, the balsamic vinegar, and salt and pepper to taste. Puree, and then slowly blend in the olive oil. Set the dressing aside.

2. In a large bowl, toss together the spinach, walnuts, feta, and the second pint of raspberries. Toss with the dressing and serve.

SUBSTITUTION: To make this dairy-free, skip the feta and use extra nuts or diced avocado instead. To make this heartier, feel free to add a protein of your choice, such as crisp tofu cubes, or roasted chicken strips.

PER SERVING (1 CUP): Calories: 269; Total fat: 19g; Sodium: 327mg; Carbohydrates: 23g; Fiber: 10g; Protein: 7g

Leafy Greens, Chickpea, and Barley Salad with Lemony Mustard Dressing

SERVES 2

PREP TIME: 15 minutes • **COOK TIME:** 25 to 40 minutes

Anemia, GI (constipation), Taste Changes

Barley is a nutritious option full of fiber, protein, and iron. Barley also offers vitamin B$_6$, a vitamin in which as many as one-third of all Americans are deficient, and is needed to form hemoglobin in the blood. It's best to use quick barley for this recipe. It's just as nutritious as longer-cooking barley, but is pre-steamed so it takes half the time.

1 cup quick-cooking barley

4 cups fresh spinach leaves,
   or mixed leafy greens

¼ cup dry roasted almonds

1 cup canned chickpeas,
   rinsed and drained

1 red, yellow, or orange
   bell pepper, diced

¼ red onion, diced

½ avocado, diced

¼ cup Lemony Mustard
   Dressing (page 136)

1. In a medium saucepan, bring 2 cups of water to a boil over high heat. Add the barley, and simmer for 25 minutes. Add more water if the pot becomes dry before the barley has finished cooking. After 25 minutes, check every 5 minutes to see if the barley has reached the desired chewiness.

2. In a medium bowl, combine the spinach, almonds, chickpeas, bell pepper, onion, and avocado. Set aside.

3. Add the Lemony Mustard dressing to the salad, and toss until well distributed.

PREP AHEAD: Make a pot of barley for the week, and add it as a dose of fiber to cold salads or warm up for a hot side dish. Store barley in an airtight glass container for 3 to 4 days in the refrigerator or up to 2 months in the freezer.

PER SERVING (1½ CUPS): Calories: 865; Total fat: 40g; Sodium: 529mg; Carbohydrates: 114g; Fiber: 28g; Protein: 23g

Chicken Tomato Hummus Sandwich

SERVES 2

PREP TIME: 10 minutes • **COOK TIME:** 15 minutes

Anemia, GI (constipation), Weight Loss

You can add nutrition to any sandwich by using hummus instead of mayonnaise. Hummus alone is an excellent option when foods are hard to chew and swallow, and really versatile because you can add different herbs and spices to change the flavor profile. This homemade version is incredibly easy to make, has more fiber and less oil, and tastes so much better than store-bought. Traditional hummus is always thinned with tahini, a sesame paste.

FOR THE HUMMUS:

1 (15-ounce) can chickpeas, drained and rinsed

2 tablespoons tahini

2 tablespoons extra-virgin olive oil

3 garlic cloves

Juice of 1 lemon

Kosher salt, optional

1 to 2 tablespoons water, if needed

FOR THE SANDWICH:

2 (4 to 5-ounce) organic boneless, skinless chicken breasts

Kosher salt, optional

Freshly ground black pepper, optional

4 slices whole wheat or sprouted bread

4 tablespoons hummus, divided

1 medium tomato, sliced into 4 slices

1. Preheat the oven to 450°F.

2. **Make the hummus:** In the bowl of a blender or food processor, combine the chickpeas, tahini, olive oil, garlic, lemon juice, and salt (if using), and pulse until smooth. Add 1 or 2 tablespoons of water at a time, if you desire a smoother texture.

3. **Make the sandwich:** Season the chicken with salt and pepper, if using. Cook the chicken on a sheet pan prepared with parchment paper in the oven for 15 minutes. While the chicken cooks, toast the bread, if you prefer. Spread 2 tablespoons of hummus each on two slices of the bread.

4. When the chicken is done, place one chicken breast on each piece of bread with hummus, and top with 2 tomato slices and the other slice of bread.

MAKE IT EVEN EASIER: You can buy prepackaged hummus at most grocery stores to save some time. You can also buy rotisserie chicken if you don't want to cook chicken. A rotisserie chicken has many uses for leftovers, such as sandwiches, salads, and a protein boost for cold meals.

PER SERVING (1 SANDWICH): Calories: 362; Total fat: 8g; Sodium: 318mg; Carbohydrates: 36g; Fiber: 6g; Protein: 35g

Arugula Beet Sweet Potato Quinoa Salad

SERVES 4

PREP AND COOLING TIME: 5 minutes and 5 minutes • **COOK TIME:** 40 minutes

Anemia, Fatigue, GI (constipation)

This simple salad offers layers of nutrition: Quinoa is rich in protein, sweet potatoes and beets provide fiber, and avocado is a healthy fat. Both the beets and arugula are powerhouses for the blood, helping to lower blood pressure and improve blood flow. Make extra beets and sweet potatoes, and use them for other meals.

3 large beets, peeled and cubed

3 large sweet potatoes,
  peeled and cubed

2 tablespoons extra-virgin olive oil

3 cups arugula

2 cups cooked quinoa

1 avocado, diced

Kosher salt

Black pepper

1. Preheat the oven to 400°F, and line a baking sheet with parchment paper.

2. Spread the beets and sweet potatoes in a single layer on the baking sheet, and drizzle with olive oil, being sure to coat each piece.

3. Roast the vegetables for 20 minutes, then flip them and roast for an additional 20 minutes, until they are slightly browned. Remove them from the oven, and let them cool for 5 minutes.

4. In a large bowl, combine the arugula, quinoa, avocado, beets, and sweet potatoes. Add salt and pepper to taste.

MAKE IT EVEN EASIER: You can buy precooked beets, vacuum packed, at some local grocery stores. Wash them to remove the red juice.

FLAVOR BOOST: Add pumpkin seeds for more protein, magnesium, and iron, or top with your favorite dressing, onion salt, or everything bagel seasoning for a flavor boost.

PER SERVING (1 CUP): Calories: 374; Total fat: 16g; Sodium: 171mg;
Carbohydrates: 52g; Fiber: 11g; Protein: 8g

Crunchy Cabbage Edamame Slaw with Dressing

SERVES 5
PREP TIME: 15 minutes

Anemia, Fatigue, Taste Changes

Soy should come with a label, "Soy does not cause breast cancer," because there is so much misinformation that accompanies this food. It's actually a fine protein replacement for meat, and filled with plant nutrients and minerals. Edamame will help meet your iron needs for the day. This salad adds mandarin oranges, both for the healing vitamin C, and to help mask flavors when foods just don't taste right.

2 teaspoons grated fresh ginger

3 tablespoons tamari sauce

¼ cup rice vinegar

2 tablespoons maple syrup

2 tablespoons sesame oil

3 cups shredded (from 1 medium) green cabbage

1 cup shredded (from ½ small) purple cabbage

1 cup frozen edamame, thawed

4 scallions, green parts, diced

1 cup shredded carrots

2 (8.25-ounce) cans mandarin oranges or 4 fresh mandarin oranges, sectioned

½ cup slivered almonds

2 tablespoons sesame seeds

1. In a small bowl or jar, mix together the ginger, tamari, vinegar, maple syrup, and sesame oil. Set the dressing aside.

2. In a large bowl, combine the green and purple cabbage, edamame, onions, carrots, oranges, almonds, and sesame seeds. Stir to combine, and toss the dressing with the salad.

3. Enjoy immediately, or let it marinate for an hour to enhance the flavors. This salad will last in the refrigerator for 3 days once dressed.

PER SERVING (1 CUP): Calories: 267; Total fat: 15g; Sodium: 523mg; Carbohydrates: 28g; Fiber: 7g; Protein: 9g

Protein, Lettuce, and Tomato Sandwich (PLT)

SERVES 4

PREP TIME: 5 minutes • **COOK TIME:** 16 minutes

Anemia, Fatigue, Taste Changes

You'll find there's no need to press tofu here, so this recipe is a quick prep for a hearty, protein-filled sandwich. The nutritional yeast adds a flavor reminiscent of Parmesan cheese, but it's filled with iron and B12 that you need during cancer treatment. Arugula adds a peppery kick, but you can substitute any leafy green.

1 (14-ounce) package extra-firm tofu
2 tablespoons extra-virgin olive oil
2 teaspoons garlic powder
2 teaspoons soy sauce
2 tablespoons nutritional yeast
Freshly ground black pepper
2 teaspoons Dijon mustard, divided

1 avocado, sliced in quarters
1 medium tomato, thinly
　sliced into quarters
1 pickle, sliced
1 cup arugula, divided
8 slices multigrain or
　sourdough bread, toasted

1. Remove the tofu from its packaging, and allow the water to drain. Stand the block upright, and slice into 4 thick slices.

2. In a large sauté pan, heat the olive oil over medium heat. Add the slices of tofu to the pan, then sprinkle the garlic powder and soy sauce over the slices. Sauté for about 8 minutes until browned, then flip gently. Add the nutritional yeast and black pepper to taste. Sauté until the other side is browned, about 8 minutes.

3. To make the sandwiches, divide and layer the mustard, avocado, tomato, pickle, and arugula on each of the 4 slices of toasted bread. Add a tofu slice to each sandwich, top each sandwich with another piece of bread, and eat immediately.

PER SERVING (1 SANDWICH): Calories: 438; Total fat: 25g; Sodium: 367mg; Carbohydrates: 34g; Fiber: 10g; Protein: 24g

Creamy Avocado Vegetable Burritos

SERVES 4

PREP TIME: 10 minutes • **COOK TIME:** 10 minutes

GI (constipation), Taste Changes, Weight Loss

Burritos are the ultimate prep-in-advance recipe. When wrapped in foil, they stay fresh in the refrigerator for a couple of days, and are easy to reheat.

1 tablespoon extra-virgin olive oil

1 yellow onion, thinly sliced

1 zucchini, diced

½ teaspoon kosher salt

½ teaspoon freshly ground black pepper

½ teaspoon ground cumin

1 (15.5-ounce) can pinto beans, drained and rinsed

½ small head cabbage, shredded

¼ cup guacamole

4 large tortillas, whole wheat or gluten-free

½ cup chopped fresh cilantro, divided

1 large avocado, quartered

1. In a large skillet, heat the oil over medium heat. Add the onion and zucchini, stirring occasionally for 5 to 7 minutes, until the vegetables soften. Add the salt, pepper, cumin, and beans and stir well to combine, cooking 1 to 2 minutes more until the bean filling is hot.

2. In a large bowl, combine the cabbage and guacamole, and stir to combine.

3. Assemble as many burritos as you can eat in 2 days. For each burrito, lay a tortilla on a flat surface and top with ¼ of the bean filling, followed by ¼ of the cabbage mixture, ¼ of the cilantro, and ¼ of the avocado on top. Wrap the burrito tightly by folding the top and bottom of the tortilla over the filling and wrapping the left and right sides so they overlap.

4. Either eat immediately or wrap the assembled burritos individually in foil, and refrigerate for up to 2 days. For the remaining components, store the bean mixture, cabbage mixture, avocado, and cilantro in separate small containers.

PER SERVING: Calories: 516; Total fat: 26g; Sodium: 404mg; Carbohydrates: 63g; Fiber: 19g; Protein: 15g;

Tofu and Veggie Skewers

SERVES 4

PREP AND MARINATING/SOAKING TIME: 5 minutes and 20 minutes
COOK TIME: 35 minutes

Anemia, GI (diarrhea), Taste Changes

In this recipe, tofu and veggies are marinated in a homemade, all-natural sauce and then oven-baked on skewers in a delicious, hands-free preparation style that's fun to eat. Serve over brown rice for a balanced, filling meal.

Garlic-Herb Marinated
  Tofu (page 132)
½ red onion, cut into large chunks
1 medium zucchini, cut
  into ½-inch slices

1 yellow squash or yellow bell
  pepper, cut into ½-inch slices
1 (8-ounce) package mushrooms,
  stems removed

1. Marinate the tofu for 20 minutes as directed in the recipe for Garlic-Herb Marinated Tofu. At the same time, soak 8 (6-inch) wooden skewers in water (so they don't char in the oven) for 20 minutes.

2. Preheat the oven to 425°F. Line a large baking sheet with parchment paper.

3. To make the skewers, slide the marinated tofu slices (reserve the marinade), chunks of onion, zucchini slices, squash slices, and mushrooms in an alternating pattern onto the skewers, leaving 1 inch of skewer empty on each end.

4. Transfer the skewers to the pan, and drizzle half of the reserved tofu marinade over them. Set the remaining marinade aside. Bake the skewers for 20 minutes, then flip them and coat with the remaining marinade. Bake for 15 to 20 minutes more, until the tofu has browned and the vegetables are soft.

PREP AHEAD: Store in the refrigerator for up to 5 days.

PER SERVING (2 SKEWERS): Calories: 210; Total fat: 13g; Sodium: 308mg; Carbohydrates: 14g; Fiber: 2g; Protein: 14g

Sweet Potato Avocado Toast

SERVES 5

PREP TIME: 10 minutes • **COOK TIME:** 20 minutes

GI (constipation), Taste Changes, Weight Loss

Maximize your vegetable intake by making "toast" out of sweet potatoes. Feel free to get creative with the toppings, adding in even more veggies.

3 large sweet potatoes, cut lengthwise into ¼-inch-thick slices
5 large eggs
3 avocados, halved and pitted
1 garlic clove, minced
1 teaspoon kosher salt

1 teaspoon freshly ground black pepper
1 teaspoon ground cumin
Juice of 1 lime
5 radishes, finely chopped

1. Preheat the oven to 400°F. Line a large baking sheet with parchment paper.

2. Arrange the sweet potato slices on the baking sheet, and bake for 20 minutes, or until tender. It's okay if they're slightly undercooked; you'll be reheating them later. Transfer them to a wire rack to cool thoroughly.

3. While the potatoes are baking, place the eggs in a pot of water so that they're completely covered. Bring to a boil over high heat. Then, remove from the heat, cover, and let stand for 11 minutes. Drain and set the eggs aside to cool.

4. While the eggs are cooling, in a large bowl, scoop the flesh from the avocados, and mash it lightly with a fork until chunky. Add the garlic, salt, pepper, cumin, lime juice, and radishes. Mix with a wooden spoon until all ingredients are incorporated.

5. To serve, reheat the slices of sweet potato in the toaster oven or oven for 4 to 5 minutes at 400°F. Spread ¼ cup of avocado mixture onto each piece of "toast." Peel and slice a hard-boiled egg and fan it out on top of the avocado mixture on top of each piece of toast.

PER SERVING (2 TOASTS): Calories: 364; Total fat: 23g; Sodium: 356mg; Carbohydrates: 32g; Fiber: 13g; Protein: 12g

Curry-Roasted Cauliflower and Chickpea Salad

SERVES 4

PREP AND COOLING TIME: 10 minutes and 5 minutes · **COOK TIME:** 15 minutes

Anemia, GI (constipation), Weight Loss

Even people who think they don't like cauliflower love it roasted. Most curry powders contain many anti-inflammatory spices such as turmeric, cumin, and fenugreek. The chickpeas add always-needed protein and fiber, creating a complete meal.

2 cups cauliflower florets

¼ cup melted coconut oil or extra-virgin olive oil

1½ teaspoons curry powder

1 teaspoon kosher salt

3 cups romaine lettuce, cut across into 1-inch ribbons

1 (15-ounce) can chickpeas, drained and rinsed

2 tablespoons freshly squeezed lime juice

2 tablespoons chopped fresh cilantro

1 tablespoon extra-virgin olive oil

¼ teaspoon freshly ground black pepper

1. Preheat the oven to 400°F.

2. In a 9-by-13-inch baking dish, toss together the cauliflower, coconut oil, curry powder, and salt until well mixed.

3. Transfer the dish to the oven, and roast until tender, about 15 minutes. Remove from the oven, and let cool to room temperature.

4. Add the lettuce, chickpeas, lime juice, cilantro, olive oil, and pepper; toss to combine, and serve.

PREP AHEAD: This salad can be made ahead of time without the lettuce and stored, covered, for several days in the refrigerator. Add the lettuce right before serving.

PER SERVING: Calories: 275; Total fat: 19g; Sodium: 603mg Carbohydrates: 23g; Fiber: 6g; Protein: 7g

Watermelon and Quinoa Salad with Feta and Mint

SERVES 4

PREP AND COOLING TIME: 5 minutes and 5 minutes · **COOK TIME:** 20 minutes

Anemia, GI (diarrhea), Taste Changes

This salad screams summer. The quinoa adds protein and fiber, and the watermelon is sweet and juicy and a delicious counterpart to the creamy feta. Choose watermelon to counter bitter, acidic, or metallic tastes. Because most markets sell precut watermelon, this salad is a breeze to create.

1 cup quinoa
1 teaspoon kosher salt
¼ cup extra-virgin olive oil
2 tablespoons freshly
  squeezed lemon juice
2 cups seeded watermelon,
  cut into ½-inch pieces

1 scallion, both white and
  green parts, thinly sliced
½ cup crumbled feta
¼ cup finely chopped fresh mint
¼ teaspoon freshly ground
  black pepper

1. In a large pot, combine the quinoa, 2 cups of water, and salt. Bring to a boil, reduce the heat to a simmer, and cook, partially covered, until all the water has been absorbed, about 20 minutes. Remove from the heat, let cool to room temperature, and fluff with a fork.

2. Once cooled, add the oil and lemon juice, and mix well. Add the watermelon and scallion, and gently mix until just combined. Sprinkle the feta, mint, and pepper over the salad, and serve. This salad is best eaten shortly after it's been made, but it can be stored, covered, in the refrigerator for 24 hours.

SUBSTITUTION: If using precooked quinoa, use 3 cups.

PER SERVING: Calories: 473; Total fat: 29g; Sodium: 1,189mg; Carbohydrates: 36g; Fiber: 4g; Protein: 19g

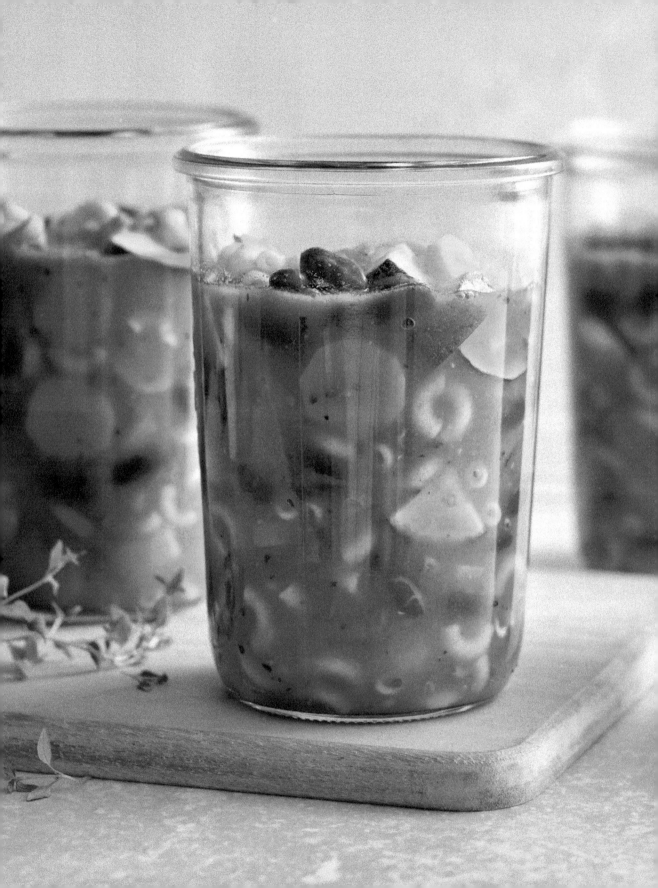

7

Soups and Stews

Potato Leek Celery Soup

SERVES 4

PREP TIME: 15 minutes • **COOK TIME:** 55 minutes

GI (diarrhea), Nausea, Swallowing (includes mouth and throat soreness)

One frustrating side effect is something called early satiety, which means that you feel full after only a few bites. To make your way around this, try more soups or broths, because liquids leave the stomach quicker. This creamy comfort soup is also a good option when you can only tolerate pureed food, but need to pack in a bit more nutrition.

2 tablespoons extra-virgin olive oil
2 leeks, sliced
4 celery stalks, chopped
4 medium Yukon Gold potatoes,
  peeled and diced

1 bay leaf
3 fresh thyme sprigs
4 cups vegetable or chicken stock
Kosher salt
Freshly ground black pepper

1. In a large saucepan, heat the olive oil over medium heat and add the leeks and celery. Cover and cook for 10 minutes, then uncover and stir for a few seconds. Add the potatoes, bay leaf, and thyme, then cover and cook for another 10 minutes.

2. Uncover the soup, and stir again. Add the stock, and bring the mixture to a boil. Reduce the heat to simmer for 30 minutes. Remove from the heat, and remove the bay leaf and thyme sprigs.

3. Use either an immersion blender or a blender to puree the soup to your desired consistency. Add salt and pepper to taste.

MAKE IT EVEN EASIER: An immersion blender is a useful tool to save time and effort for soups and smoothies. If you use a blender, you will have to remove the soup from the saucepan, and, depending on the size of your blender, you may have to do it in two rounds.

PER SERVING (1 CUP): Calories: 374; Total fat: 7g; Sodium: 190mg; Carbohydrates: 71g; Fiber: 9g; Protein: 8g

Pumpkin Soup

SERVES 6

PREP TIME: 5 minutes · **COOK TIME:** 15 minutes

Nausea, Swallowing (includes mouth and throat soreness), Weight Loss

Soup is a valuable way of obtaining nutrients and combating side effects during treatments. In the fall, you can easily find fresh pumpkin, but in the interest of time, use the canned version. The bright orange color is your cue to the high amount of beta-carotene, a cancer fighter. This soup can be frozen in large ice cube (portion-sized) trays with lids, or in a large airtight container, for up to 3 months.

1 tablespoon extra-virgin olive oil

1 yellow onion, chopped

1 quart low-sodium chicken broth or vegetable broth

2 (15-ounce) cans pumpkin puree

½ teaspoon dried cumin

½ teaspoon dried ginger

Kosher salt

Freshly ground black pepper

1. In a stockpot or Dutch oven, heat the oil over medium heat. Add the onion and sauté until soft and beginning to brown, about 5 minutes. Add the chicken broth, pumpkin, cumin, ginger, and salt and pepper to taste. Bring to a simmer for 5 to 10 minutes.

2. Remove from the heat, cool, then use an immersion blender to blend until smooth. (Alternatively, transfer in batches to a blender and then back to the stockpot.)

3. Return the heat to medium, and warm the soup through. Serve immediately.

FLAVOR BOOST: If you desire a creamier or heartier recipe, add 1 cup of coconut milk to this soup with the chicken stock. Full-fat Greek yogurt also makes a great topping, as long as you're not feeling nauseous; fat can make nausea worse.

PER SERVING (1 CUP): Calories: 80; Total fat: 3g; Sodium: 203mg; Carbohydrates: 14g; Fiber: 5g; Protein: 2g

Hot and Sour Soup

SERVES 2

PREP TIME: 10 minutes • **COOKS TIME:** 25 minutes

Taste Changes, Weight Loss

Vinegar and spices hide off flavors; add as much as needed to foods that are now flavorless. This hot and sour soup was a bowl of comfort to me in treatment.

1 (15-ounce) can reduced-sodium vegetable broth

1 package fresh shiitake mushrooms, stems removed and thinly sliced

1 teaspoon freshly grated ginger

2 cups finely chopped bok choy

½ (8-ounce) can bamboo shoots

1 teaspoon hot chili sauce, or to taste

1 tablespoon rice wine vinegar

1 teaspoon reduced-sodium soy sauce

1 tablespoon cornstarch

1 cup thinly sliced extra-firm tofu

1 scallion, green parts only, finely chopped

1 teaspoon sesame oil

1. In a large saucepan, bring the broth to a boil. Add the mushrooms, and boil for 2 minutes. Reduce the heat to a simmer and add the ginger, bok choy, and bamboo shoots. Simmer for 4 minutes. Add the chili sauce, vinegar, and soy sauce. Simmer 3 minutes more.

2. While the broth is simmering, mix the cornstarch and ¼ cup water in a glass measuring cup.

3. Add the tofu to the saucepan, and simmer for 10 minutes. Add the cornstarch mixture and stir for 2 to 3 minutes.

4. Remove the saucepan from the heat, add the scallion and sesame oil, and serve.

SUBSTITUTION: For more protein, add a cooked egg white to each portion.

PER SERVING (1 CUP): Calories: 184; Total fat: 9g; Sodium: 116mg; Carbohydrates: 17g; Fiber: 5g; Protein: 14g

Creamy Nutmeg Cauliflower Soup

SERVES 4 TO 6

PREP TIME: 10 minutes • **COOK TIME:** 30 to 40 minutes

GI (constipation), Nausea, Swallowing

When you want something light but heartier than broth, this creamy soup will work. Plus, this soup only gets better (thicker) as it chills, and cold or room-temperature foods are a relief for mouth soreness. It can also be served cold for nausea or when cooking smells are bothersome.

2 tablespoons extra-virgin olive oil	¼ teaspoon black pepper
1 large sweet onion, chopped	6 cups vegetable broth
1 russet potato, peeled and chopped	1 dash nutmeg
1 large head cauliflower, chopped	Grated zest of 1 small lemon
1 teaspoon kosher salt	

1. In a large saucepan, heat the olive oil over medium heat, and then sauté the onion and potato until the onion is translucent, about 3 to 5 minutes. Add the cauliflower, salt, and pepper. Cook for 3 more minutes. Add the vegetable broth, and bring the soup to a boil. Reduce the heat, cover, and simmer for 20 to 30 minutes, until the potato and cauliflower are soft enough to be mashed.

2. Puree the soup using an immersion blender (or in a blender or food processor, 2 cups at a time, and then transfer back to the saucepan).

3. Bring the blended soup to a simmer, just until bubbles begin to break the surface. Add the nutmeg and zest. Serve hot or chill for several hours and serve cold.

SUBSTITUTION: Replace one of the cups of broth with a cup of unsweetened, unflavored soy milk. This lends more creaminess to the soup without dairy fat, and adds a protein boost. You can also try a plant-based, unflavored half-and-half. Use ½ cup instead of the equivalent broth.

PER SERVING (1 CUP): Calories: 212; Total fat: 7g; Sodium: 365mg; Carbohydrates: 33g; Fiber: 6g; Protein: 7g

Matzo Ball Soup

SERVES 6
PREP AND CHILLING TIME: 20 minutes and 15 minutes
COOK TIME: 1 hour and 10 minutes

GI (diarrhea), Nausea, Swallowing (includes mouth and throat soreness)

You didn't think we would have recipes for recovery without matzo ball soup, did you? This broth is suitable for so many side effects, it's no wonder it has stood the test of time. You may need low fiber after different types of surgery, and low fat for nausea and digestive difficulties. Homemade matzo balls are ideal, because you can control the sodium. A bowl of broth can be added throughout the day for more nutrition.

FOR THE MATZO BALLS:

1 cup matzo meal
2 eggs
½ cup water

1 teaspoon kosher salt
1 tsp ground turmeric

FOR THE SOUP:

1 yellow onion, sliced thin
3 garlic cloves, minced
2 tablespoons extra-virgin olive oil
3 (6-ounce) boneless, skinless
   chicken breasts, coarsely chopped
3 celery stalks, sliced thin
2 parsnips, peeled, sliced thin
3 carrots, sliced thin

3 quarts chicken broth
1 teaspoon dried thyme
1 teaspoon dried parsley
2 bay leaves
½ teaspoon celery seed
Kosher salt
Freshly ground black pepper

1. **Make the matzo balls**: In a medium mixing bowl, combine the matzo meal, eggs, water, salt, and turmeric. Mix together until all water is absorbed and the mixture forms a paste-like dough. Let the mixture chill for 15 to 20 minutes in the refrigerator. Alternatively, freeze the matzo mixture in greased ice cube trays.

2. **Make the soup**: In a large pot, heat the onion, garlic, and olive oil over medium heat. Sauté until the onion is translucent. Add the chicken, celery, parsnips, and carrots. Sauté until the chicken is thoroughly cooked, about 12 minutes.

3. Add the chicken broth along with the thyme, parsley, bay leaves, and celery seed to the pot. Add salt and pepper to taste, and bring the soup to a boil.

4. Allow the soup to boil for 10 minutes, then reduce to a simmer. Remove the matzo mixture from refrigerator. Drop by teaspoonfuls into the soup pot. If using the frozen mixture, release matzo cubes with a spoon and drop into the soup pot.

5. Cover the pot, and reduce to a medium simmer. Allow the matzo balls to simmer at least 40 minutes, then serve.

SUBSTITUTION: You can leave out the chicken breast if you choose and use vegetarian broth. You can add 1 cup of pasta or white rice, or add 1 medium potato, diced, if you want the soup to be heartier.

PREP AHEAD: The soup and the matzo balls can be frozen for up to 3 months in a reusable storage bag or glass container. To reheat, boil water, and drop the matzo balls in gently.

PER SERVING (1 CUP): Calories: 300; Total fat: 8g; Sodium: 489mg; Carbohydrates: 33g; Fiber: 3g; Protein: 24g

Minestrone with Herbs and Whole-Grain Pasta

SERVES 6

PREP TIME: 10 minutes • **COOK TIME:** 45 minutes

Anemia, GI (constipation), Taste Changes

When your appetite is better, embrace it and try to eat more nourishing foods. Filling bean soups are a vehicle for nutrition and comfort, all in one bowl. This Italian-inspired soup has a variety of antioxidant-packed veggies and whole-grain pasta. Kidney beans offer protein and also boost iron, which may help with fatigue. The umami flavor found in tomatoes can mask unpleasant taste changes from treatment.

2 tablespoons extra-virgin olive oil

½ yellow onion, diced

1 large carrot, cut into thin rounds

1 cup green beans, trimmed and cut into thirds

1 medium zucchini, halved lengthwise and cut crosswise into ¼-inch half-moons

2 garlic cloves, minced

1 teaspoon dried basil

1 teaspoon dried oregano

1 teaspoon kosher salt

1 teaspoon freshly ground black pepper

1 (14.5-ounce) can diced tomatoes

4 cups vegetable broth

1 (15-ounce) can kidney beans, drained and rinsed

1 cup whole wheat or bean rotini or elbow pasta

1. In a large pot, warm the olive oil over medium-high heat. Add the onion, carrot, green beans, and zucchini, and cook for 10 to 12 minutes, or until the onion is translucent and the vegetables soften. Add the garlic, basil, oregano, salt, and pepper, and cook for another 1 to 2 minutes, stirring frequently.

2. Add the tomatoes and broth. Increase the heat to medium-high, and bring the soup to a boil; then cover, reduce the heat to medium-low, and let simmer for 15 minutes.

3. Add the beans and uncooked pasta, and cook, uncovered, for 11 to 15 minutes more, until the pasta is tender. Serve immediately or portion the soup into 6 servings and let it cool it before freezing. It will last in the refrigerator for up to 3 days, or in the freezer for up to 2 months.

FLAVOR BOOST: This soup also tastes great prepared spicy—just add ½ teaspoon red pepper flakes. Other herbs, such as fresh basil, fresh dill, thyme, or a bay leaf (removed when the soup is done), also enhance the flavor of this recipe and provide antioxidants.

PER SERVING: Calories: 161; Total fat: 5g; Sodium: 287mg; Carbohydrates: 25g; Fiber: 6g; Protein: 6g

Turkey Taco Soup

SERVES 4 TO 6

PREP TIME: 15 minutes • **COOK TIME:** 20 minutes

GI (constipation), Taste Changes, Weight Loss

This hearty, health-supportive soup can be put together in minutes. Feel free to add or remove ingredients as you like; if you don't like beans, you can omit those. Layering a variety of textures can counter unwelcome taste changes. Serve this hearty soup with yogurt on top, and the coolness will contrast with the hot soup. You can also top with chopped scallions or fresh cilantro.

1 tablespoon extra-virgin
  olive oil
1 pound ground turkey
1 zucchini, sliced
2 garlic cloves, minced
1 teaspoon kosher salt
1 teaspoon chipotle powder
½ teaspoon ground cumin

¼ teaspoon freshly ground
  black pepper
1 (15-ounce) can black beans,
  drained and rinsed
1 (14.5-ounce) can diced fire-roasted
  with their juices, optional
1 cup frozen corn, optional
4 cups chicken or vegetable broth

1. In a Dutch oven, heat the oil over high heat. Add the ground turkey and cook, stirring frequently until browned, about 5 minutes.

2. Add the zucchini, garlic, salt, chipotle powder, cumin, and pepper, and sauté until tender, about 5 minutes. Add the black beans, fire-roasted tomatoes (if using), corn (if using), and broth. Bring it to a boil, then reduce to a simmer to heat through and combine the flavors, about 10 minutes.

3. Ladle into bowls and serve.

SUBSTITUTION: To make this soup vegan, substitute a 15-ounce can of kidney beans, drained and rinsed, for the turkey, and use vegetable broth.

PER SERVING (SOUP ONLY): Calories: 370; Total fat: 14g; Sodium: 1,020mg; Carbohydrates: 33g; Fiber: 10g; Protein: 29g

Lentil Stew

SERVES 4 TO 6

PREP TIME: 15 minutes • **COOK TIME:** 15 minutes

Anemia, GI (constipation), Swallowing (includes mouth and throat soreness)

Most stews take hours to cook, but this restorative dish, perfect for dinner or lunch, cooks up quickly. There's nothing like a hearty stew to take the chill off in cold winter months. This plant-based recipe is loaded with nutritious anti-inflammatory power foods, protein, and iron.

1 tablespoon extra-virgin olive oil
1 onion, chopped
3 carrots, sliced
8 Brussels sprouts, halved
1 large turnip, peeled, quartered, and sliced
1 garlic clove, sliced
6 cups vegetable broth

1 (15-ounce) can lentils, drained and rinsed
1 cup frozen corn
1 teaspoon kosher salt
¼ teaspoon freshly ground black pepper
1 tablespoon chopped fresh parsley

1. In a Dutch oven, heat the oil over high heat. Add the onion, and sauté until softened, about 3 minutes. Add the carrots, Brussels sprouts, turnip, and garlic, and sauté for an additional 3 minutes.

2. Add the broth, and bring to a boil. Reduce to a simmer, and cook until the vegetables are tender, about 5 minutes. Add the lentils, corn, salt, pepper, and parsley, and cook for an additional minute to heat the lentils and corn. Serve hot.

SUBSTITUTION: This stew is as versatile as it is simple. Feel free to use any beans or vegetables you have; it's a great way to use up leftover vegetables at the end of the week. Store in a covered container in the refrigerator for 3 to 4 days, or in the freezer for up to 2 months.

PER SERVING: Calories: 240; Total fat: 4g; Sodium: 870mg; Carbohydrates: 42g; Fiber: 12g; Protein: 10g

Roasted Butternut Squash Soup with Sage

SERVES 4

PREP TIME: 10 minutes • **COOK TIME:** 10 minutes

GI (diarrhea), Taste Changes, Weight Loss

Winter squash and sage are two flavors that go well together. A topping of yogurt and pomegranate seeds rounds out this mouthwatering dish for a flavor punch when appetite lags. Omit the pomegranate seeds if you have difficulty swallowing.

2 tablespoons extra-virgin olive oil
2 shallots, finely chopped
1 garlic clove, minced
2 cups butternut squash
  (or pumpkin) puree
2 cups vegetable or chicken broth
½ cup unsweetened coconut
  milk, optional

1 teaspoon kosher salt
¼ teaspoon freshly ground
  black pepper
8 fresh sage leaves
⅓ cup pomegranate seeds
¼ cup plain Greek yogurt, optional

1. In a Dutch oven, heat the oil over medium-high heat. Add the shallots and garlic, and sauté until softened, 3 to 5 minutes. Add the butternut squash and broth, and stir to combine.

2. Bring to a boil, reduce to a simmer, and cook for 3 to 5 minutes to heat through. Add the coconut milk (if using), and season with salt and pepper.

3. Garnish with the sage leaves, pomegranate seeds, and yogurt (if using), and serve.

PREP AHEAD: Store leftover soup in a covered container in the refrigerator for up to 3 to 4 days or in the freezer for 2 months.

SUBSTITUTION: If you can't find pomegranate seeds, try dried cranberries.

PER SERVING (INCLUDING COCONUT MILK AND YOGURT): Calories: 200; Total fat: 16g; Sodium: 820mg; Carbohydrates: 11g; Fiber: 2g; Protein: 4g

"Eat Your Greens" Soup

SERVES 4

PREP TIME: 10 minutes · **COOK TIME:** 20 minutes

Anemia, Swallowing (includes mouth and throat soreness), Weight Loss

Sip this broth throughout the day when you need nourishment but can't stomach an entire meal. This recipe uses kale, Swiss chard, and mustard greens for iron and calcium. Check with your medical team if you're on blood thinners, because this amount of vitamin K from the greens may be too much to consume at once.

¼ cup extra-virgin olive oil

2 leeks, white parts only, thinly sliced

1 fennel bulb, trimmed
  and thinly sliced

1 garlic clove, peeled

1 bunch Swiss chard,
  coarsely chopped

4 cups coarsely chopped kale

4 cups coarsely chopped
  mustard greens

3 cups vegetable broth

2 tablespoons apple cider vinegar

1 teaspoon kosher salt

¼ teaspoon freshly ground
  black pepper

¼ cup chopped cashews, optional

1. In a large pot, heat the oil over high heat. Add the leeks, fennel, and garlic, and sauté until softened, about 5 minutes. Add the Swiss chard, kale, and mustard greens, and sauté until the greens wilt, 2 to 3 minutes.

2. Add the broth, and bring to a boil. Reduce the heat to a simmer, and cook until the vegetables are completely soft and tender, about 5 minutes. Stir in the vinegar, salt, pepper, and cashews (if using).

3. Using an immersion blender (or a food processor or blender in batches), puree the soup in the pot until smooth, and serve warm.

FLAVOR BOOST: This soup makes a great base soup to add all kinds of wonderful things, such as cooked chicken, fish, or beans.

PER SERVING: Calories: 238; Total fat: 14g; Sodium: 1,294mg; Carbohydrates: 22g; Fiber: 6g; Protein: 9g

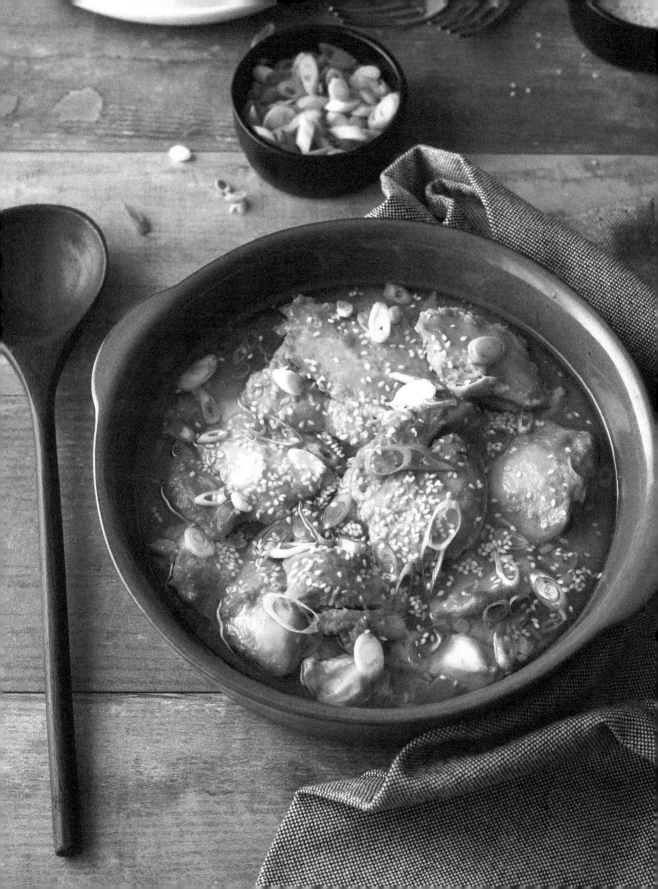

8

Fortifying Meals

Tuscan Chicken Skillet

SERVES 6

PREP TIME: 5 minutes · **COOK TIME:** 30 minutes

Fatigue, GI (constipation), Weight Loss

This dish cooks up faster than roasted chicken, when you need a hearty meal. To cope with a variety of taste changes, use layers of flavor. Strong flavors are needed to mask bitter and metallic tastes. Tomatoes disguise a too-salty taste, and, to reduce sodium further, rinse the canned beans, which removes more than 90 percent of the sodium. Add broth to make it easier to chew and swallow; you can also dip bread into the sauce to soften it.

3 tablespoons extra-virgin olive oil, divided

6 (4 to 5-ounce) organic boneless, skinless chicken breasts

Kosher salt

Freshly ground black pepper

2 (10-ounce containers) white mushrooms, sliced

1 white onion, chopped

1⅓ cup sun-dried tomatoes

6 garlic cloves, minced

2 (14.5-ounce) cans diced fire-roasted tomatoes

2 (15-ounce) cans white kidney beans

2 tablespoons dried oregano

2 tablespoons dried thyme

Fresh parsley for garnish, optional

1. In a large skillet, heat 2 tablespoons of olive oil over medium heat, and add the chicken breasts, sprinkled with salt and pepper to taste, if desired. Cook for 4 to 5 minutes on each side, then set the chicken aside on a plate.

2. In the same skillet, sauté the mushrooms for 4 minutes. Set them aside. Put the third tablespoon of olive oil in the skillet, and add the onion, sun-dried tomatoes, and garlic. Sauté for 4 minutes.

3. Add the fire-roasted tomatoes, white kidney beans, oregano, and thyme. Stir them together for 1 minute. Put the chicken back in the skillet, cover, and heat over medium-low for 12 minutes. For food safety, make sure the internal temperature of the chicken reaches 165°F.

4. Add the sautéed mushrooms, turn off the heat, and garnish with fresh parsley (if using).

FLAVOR BOOST: To make the meal more delicious and even heartier, serve over white rice, brown rice, or wild rice. If you're monitoring your blood sugar, note that this addition will increase the amount of carbohydrates.

SUBSTITUTION: Make this vegetarian by omitting the chicken and adding 2 cups of cooked quinoa. The quinoa and beans in this recipe add more than enough protein to match the chicken breasts. If you can't tolerate beans right now, substitute sautéed crumbled tofu instead. This will resemble more of a stew, and you can add vegetable broth as needed.

PER SERVING (1 CHICKEN BREAST): Calories: 464; Total fat: 11g; Sodium: 272mg; Carbohydrates: 50g; Fiber: 15g; Protein: 44g

Tofu with Buckwheat Soba Noodles and Vegetables

SERVES 8

PREP, PRESSING, AND COOLING TIME: 10 minutes, 15 minutes, and 5 minutes
COOK TIME: 30 minutes

Fatigue, Nausea, Taste Changes

The distinctive flavors in this dish will make you forget that it's meatless. The spices also mask unpleasant flavors that might reduce your appetite. A cup of tofu contains nearly an entire meal's worth of protein, depending on your needs. The buckwheat soba noodles are chewy and provide more texture to meals when food doesn't taste the same.

2 (14-ounce) packages firm
  or extra-firm tofu
2 tablespoons grated fresh ginger
4 medium garlic cloves, minced
4 tablespoons tamari or soy sauce
4 teaspoons toasted sesame oil
2 tablespoons rice vinegar

2 teaspoons packed dark brown sugar
1 teaspoon red pepper flakes
½ cup water
12 ounces buckwheat soba noodles
4 medium heads baby
  bok choy, chopped
2 large carrots, thinly sliced

1. Preheat the oven to 400°F.

2. Wrap each block of tofu in 2 large paper towels. Place something heavy on top to press them for 15 minutes. (This step will make the tofu crispier.) Line a baking sheet with parchment paper. Cube the tofu and place it on the parchment paper in a single layer. If you need a second sheet that is fine, but make sure all the pieces are in a single layer. Bake for 30 minutes.

3. While it's baking, in the bowl of a blender, combine the ginger, garlic, tamari, sesame oil, vinegar, brown sugar, red pepper, and water, and blend until smooth, about 30 seconds. Set aside.

4. Bring a large pot of water to a boil. Add the noodles, and cook according to the package directions. Two minutes before the noodles are done, add the bok choy and carrots to the water, and simmer for 2 minutes.

5. Drain the noodles and vegetables. Remove the tofu from the oven, and let it cool for 5 minutes. Toss the noodles, tofu, and ginger garlic sauce together, and serve.

SUBSTITUTION: You can use spaghetti or ramen noodles instead of soba, or regular noodles instead of buckwheat if you choose. Egg noodles have less fiber than the other options but a good amount of protein, and are a flavorful option for GI difficulties, such as diarrhea.

PER SERVING (1 CUP): Calories: 286; Total fat: 8g; Sodium: 876mg; Carbohydrates: 40g; Fiber: 2g; Protein: 18g

Edamame Spaghetti with Turkey Meatballs

SERVES 8

PREP AND COOLING TIME: 20 minutes and 5 minutes • **COOK TIME:** 1 hour

Fatigue, GI (constipation), Swallowing (includes mouth and throat soreness)

Edamame pasta may be new to you, but it's high in protein and lower in carbohydrates than regular pasta. If you're not used to high-fiber foods, start with a small portion. The turkey meatballs can be frozen and reheated for up to three months, then added to a meal for extra flavor and protein. Add a boost of iron with a sprinkle of nutritional yeast over the finished dish. If you haven't tried nutritional yeast, it provides a cheesy taste without any dairy or fat.

FOR THE MEATBALLS:

8 cups fresh spinach

7 to 8 garlic cloves

2 tablespoons extra-virgin olive oil

Kosher salt

Freshly ground black pepper

2 (16-ounce) packages 93% lean ground turkey

FOR THE PASTA:

2 (8-ounce) packages edamame pasta   2 (16-ounce) jars marinara sauce

1. **Make the meatballs:** Preheat the oven to 350°F. Cover a medium-sized baking sheet with parchment paper, and set it aside.

2. In the bowl of a food processor, combine the spinach, garlic, and olive oil. Process these items until smooth; it may take several rounds. Add salt and pepper to taste.

3. In a large bowl, mix the raw turkey and the spinach mixture until it is completely blended. Form the mixture into 2-inch balls, and place them close together on the baking sheet. Cook them for 30 minutes, turn them, and cook them for 30 more minutes. Make sure the meatballs reach an internal temperature of 165°F. Let the meatballs cool for 5 minutes.

4. **Make the pasta**: Cook the edamame pasta per the package directions. When the pasta is done, add the marinara sauce and the meatballs and serve.

FLAVOR BOOST: Feel free to add other seasonings, such as oregano, onion powder, Italian seasoning, or fresh basil. Sprinkle some Parmesan cheese on top.

PER SERVING (1 CUP): Calories: 658; Total fat: 20g; Sodium: 660mg; Carbohydrates: 52g; Fiber: 36g; Protein: 68g

Wild Salmon and Garlic Broccoli Cooked in Ghee

MAKES 4 SERVINGS
PREP TIME: 5 minutes • **COOK TIME:** 15 minutes

Fatigue, Taste Changes, Weight Loss

A nutritious meal is possible with little effort. You can use a regular skillet with a lid here if you don't have cast iron. Salmon (sockeye especially) offers omega-3 fatty acids, found to be extremely beneficial for more advanced cancers during chemotherapy. These types of fats specifically help maintain weight and muscle during treatment. Ghee is simply butter with the water and milk solids removed for a richer flavor, and is another source of omega-3s.

2 tablespoons ghee, divided

4 (6-ounce) pieces wild sockeye salmon

Kosher salt

Freshly ground black pepper

4 cups chopped broccoli

4 to 5 garlic cloves, finely sliced

1 to 2 tablespoons chopped fresh parsley (optional)

1. In a large cast-iron skillet, melt 1 teaspoon of ghee over medium heat. Let it melt down a bit, then add the salmon and salt and pepper to taste. Cover, and cook for 3 to 4 minutes. Flip the salmon, and cook for 3 to 4 more minutes. Then remove the salmon from the skillet and transfer it to a plate.

2. In the same skillet, melt the other tablespoon of ghee, and add the broccoli. Toss the broccoli around a bit until it is coated in ghee, sprinkle with salt and pepper to taste, cover, and cook for 2 minutes.

3. Remove the lid, and add the garlic and a little more salt and pepper, if you desire. Toss again and let it cook 2 more minutes. Turn the stove off, and let it cool a bit before adding it to the plate with the salmon. Garnish with fresh parsley (if using).

FLAVOR BOOST: Add a baked sweet potato or ½ cup cooked brown rice for added satiety. Or add a tablespoon of pesto (or Tofu-Basil Sauce, page 137) for a stronger flavor.

PER SERVING (1 SALMON FILLET): Calories: 337; Total fat: 17g; Sodium: 367mg; Carbohydrates: 7g; Fiber: 2g; Protein: 39g

Lentil Walnut Zoodle Pasta

SERVES 8

PREP TIME: 20 minutes • **COOK TIME:** 45 minutes

Anemia, GI (constipation), Swallowing

This recipe will encourage you to discover new plant foods that are just as satisfying as meat. This sauce is reminiscent of a Bolognese sauce, but in this recipe, lentils are used for a meaty flavor with a boost of iron. Anemia can be common during treatments, and walnuts add more iron and protein, too. To make this sauce easier to chew and swallow, grind the walnuts in a food processor until they resemble ground meat.

1 yellow onion, chopped

4 garlic cloves, minced

1 medium carrot, finely shredded

2 tablespoons extra-virgin olive oil

⅓ cup finely chopped raw walnuts

1 cup brown canned lentils, drained and rinsed

1 (28-ounce) can crushed or diced tomatoes, with juice

3 tablespoons tomato paste

⅓ cup red wine

½ teaspoon red pepper flakes

½ teaspoon freshly ground black pepper

¼ teaspoon kosher salt

6 medium zucchini, unpeeled (or 6 cups prepackaged zoodles)

1 cup chopped fresh basil

Nutritional yeast, optional

1. In a food processor, combine the, onion, garlic, and carrots. Pulse until finely chopped, but stop before the mixture gets mushy.

2. In a large skillet, heat the olive oil over medium-low heat, add the onion, garlic, and carrot mixture, and add the chopped walnuts. Cook for 25 minutes, stirring frequently.

3. To the same skillet, add the lentils, crushed tomatoes, tomato paste, red wine, red pepper flakes, black pepper, and salt. Stir well, and cover. Simmer for 10 to 15 minutes, stirring occasionally, until the sauce is thickened and the lentils are tender.

4. While the sauce is cooking, if you're using whole zucchini, trim the ends, then make them into noodles using a spiralizer or julienne peeler. Add about half the zucchini noodles (3 cups) at a time to the skillet with the sauce. Cook in the sauce for 1 to 2 minutes, tossing continuously with tongs, until soft. Serve warm, topped with basil and nutritional yeast, if desired, for a parmigiana-like boost.

SUBSTITUTION: Use spaghetti instead of zoodles.

PREP AHEAD: Cook sauce but don't add zoodles. Freeze the sauce for up to 3 months. You can defrost and use the sauce over rice, pasta, or zoodles.

PER SERVING (1 CUP): Calories: 156; Total fat: 7g; Sodium: 175mg; Carbohydrates: 18g; Fiber: 6g; Protein: 6g

Roasted Whitefish

SERVES 8
PREP AND SOAKING TIME: 10 minutes and 12 minutes
COOK TIME: 40 minutes

GI (constipation), Nausea, Taste Changes

Baked fish works better than meat when mild nausea hits. Between the steroids and nausea from chemo, my appetite flip-flopped for days after treatment. Head off symptoms with medications; don't wait for them to rear their ugly head. Then choose the right foods and drink water in small sips. Get plenty of rest, and eat small meals throughout the day. This dish provides an optimal amount of protein and flavor. Finish with lemon wedges to amp up tartness and stimulate saliva for a dry mouth.

2 cups sun-dried tomatoes
6 (15-ounce) cans white kidney
   beans, rinsed and drained
2 bunches collard greens, thinly sliced
4 medium shallots, thinly
   sliced, divided
4 teaspoons dried thyme

⅔ cup extra-virgin olive oil, divided
8 (4- to 6-ounce) pieces
   skinless whitefish
Sea salt
Freshly ground black pepper
Lemon wedges for serving, optional

1. Preheat the oven to 350°F.

2. In a small bowl, combine the sun-dried tomatoes with 2 cups of hot water, and set aside for 12 minutes.

3. In a shallow 5- to 6-quart baking dish, combine the white kidney beans, collard greens, sun-dried tomatoes (and the hot water), half of the sliced shallot, and the thyme. Drizzle with 4 tablespoons of the olive oil. Stir to combine.

4. Arrange the fish in the dish, and season with salt and pepper to taste. Scatter the remaining shallots over the fish and beans, and pour the remaining olive oil over the top.

5. Cover with aluminum foil, and bake for 25 minutes. Remove the foil, and bake for 15 minutes longer, or until the fish is fully cooked. The internal temperature of the fish should be 145°F. Serve with lemon wedges, if desired.

SUBSTITUTION: To make this dish vegan, remove the fish and use baked tofu, or just add more beans. Squeeze lemon wedges to add flavor, or use other spices, such as oregano or dried basil.

PER SERVING (1 PIECE OF FISH): Calories: 548; Total fat: 20g; Sodium: 357mg; Carbohydrates: 56g; Fiber: 16g; Protein: 39g

Lemon-Artichoke Risotto

SERVES 5

PREP TIME: 15 minutes • **COOK TIME:** 45 minutes

GI (diarrhea), Nausea, Swallowing (includes mouth and throat soreness)

This simple, prep-friendly risotto is a great way to enjoy a rich rice dish filled with anti-inflammatory herbs and vegetables, including delicate artichokes, bright lemon, and fragrant mint. This vegan recipe needs no dairy to achieve its creamy texture. For even more protein, add cooked chicken, shrimp, or tofu. Omit the vegetables and use leftover creamy risotto anytime nausea or diarrhea develops.

4 cups vegetable broth

4 tablespoons extra-virgin
  olive oil, divided

1 (14-ounce) can or jar
  artichoke hearts, drained
  and cut into quarters

4 ounces sugar snap peas,
  trimmed and cut in half

½ medium onion, diced

1½ cups arborio rice

½ teaspoon kosher salt

¼ cup chopped fresh chives

¼ cup chopped fresh mint

½ teaspoon freshly ground
  black pepper

Juice of ½ lemon

⅓ cup chopped fresh flat-leaf parsley

1. In a large pot, bring the broth to a low simmer over medium heat. Once it's warm, remove it from the heat and set aside.

2. Meanwhile, in a large skillet, heat 2 tablespoons of oil over medium heat. Add the artichoke hearts, snap peas, and onion, and cook, stirring occasionally, for 6 to 8 minutes, until the artichoke has begun to brown and the onion is soft and translucent. Transfer the mixture to a small bowl and set aside.

3. In the same skillet, heat the remaining 2 tablespoons of oil over medium heat. Add the rice and salt, and stir to coat the rice. Cook the mixture for 2 to 3 minutes, stirring constantly; the rice may start to sizzle or crackle.

4. Reduce the heat to medium-low, then add the broth, 1 cup at a time, stirring after each cup until the liquid is absorbed (5 to 8 minutes per cup). Continue stirring so that the risotto becomes thick and creamy, 20 to 30 minutes total. Taste the risotto to ensure the grains are not too firm, and if it needs to cook longer, add up to 1 cup of water, 1/3 cup at a time, and stir until the liquid is absorbed.

5. Once the risotto is finished cooking and the liquid is absorbed, stir in the chives, mint, pepper, and the artichoke heart mixture. Once that's incorporated, add the lemon juice and parsley. Serve warm.

PREP AHEAD: Store the risotto in the refrigerator, or freeze it for up to 3 months. To serve from the refrigerator, reheat in the microwave for 1 to 2 minutes, and stir. For frozen risotto, thaw in the refrigerator overnight before reheating.

SUBSTITUTION: Add different herbs to switch things up—replace the chives with scallions, use fresh basil instead of mint, or try cilantro instead of parsley. Dried herbs can be substituted for fresh ones. Use 1 teaspoon each of basil and parsley. If you don't have fresh snap peas, you can add 1/2 cup frozen peas instead.

PER SERVING: Calories: 430; Total fat: 14g; Sodium: 164mg; Carbohydrates: 68g; Fiber: 6g; Protein: 7g

Butternut Squash, Spinach, and White Bean Enchiladas

SERVES 4

PREP TIME: 20 minutes · **COOK TIME:** 40 minutes

Anemia, GI (constipation), Taste Changes

Enchiladas definitely make great comfort food, but they also provide necessary iron when treatments affect red blood cells. You'll often feel tired from this side effect because red blood cells carry oxygen throughout the body. This recipe is also prepared with anti-inflammatory plant foods, including squash, spinach, and beans.

3 cups enchilada sauce, divided

2 tablespoons extra-virgin
 olive oil

1 small red onion, diced

2 garlic cloves, minced

1 cup cubed butternut squash

3 tablespoons water, as needed

1 teaspoon ground cumin

½ teaspoon kosher salt

½ teaspoon freshly ground
 black pepper

5 cups baby spinach

1 (15-ounce) can white beans,
 drained and rinsed

1 cup shredded Jack cheese, divided

8 (8-inch) whole wheat
 or corn tortillas

½ cup chopped fresh cilantro

1. Preheat the oven to 400°F.

2. In a 9-by-12-inch glass baking dish, pour ⅓ cup of enchilada sauce to cover the bottom evenly in a thin layer. Set aside.

3. In a large skillet, heat the oil over medium heat. Add the onion, garlic, and butternut squash, stirring occasionally for 5 to 7 minutes, or until the vegetables soften. If the mixture is starting to caramelize, add water a tablespoon at a time to prevent sticking. Add the cumin and stir to incorporate, then cover. Let the mixture continue to cook, stirring occasionally for 3 to 4 minutes more, or until the squash can be pierced easily with a fork.

4. When the squash is soft, sprinkle the mixture with the salt and pepper, then add the spinach. Cook, stirring occasionally, for 3 to 5 minutes, or until the spinach is wilted and incorporated.

5. Remove from the heat, and transfer the filling to a large bowl. Add the beans and ½ cup of cheese, and stir to incorporate.

6. Place one tortilla at a time on a cutting board or clean surface. Pour ½ cup of filling mixture into the middle, then top with ¼ cup of enchilada sauce. Carefully fold the tortilla around the filling so that the edges overlap slightly. Place the filled tortilla seam-side down into the prepared baking dish. Repeat with the remaining tortillas, setting them in a row to fill the dish completely.

7. Pour the remaining enchilada sauce on top of the prepared enchiladas, and sprinkle the remaining ½ cup of cheese evenly over the top. Bake for 20 to 30 minutes, or until the enchiladas are bubbling hot and golden brown on the edges. Remove from the oven, and let cool. Sprinkle with the cilantro, and serve.

PREP AHEAD: Store in the refrigerator for up to 5 days or in the freezer for up to 2 months. To serve, microwave the enchiladas for 1 to 2 minutes or until heated through (defrosting first, if necessary).

SUBSTITUTION: This recipe can easily be made gluten-free by using corn tortillas and choosing a gluten-free enchilada sauce. To make it dairy-free, use a nondairy cheese.

PER SERVING (2 ENCHILADAS): Calories: 601; Total fat: 33g; Sodium: 1,421mg; Carbohydrates: 64g; Fiber: 15g; Protein: 21g

Sesame Miso Chicken

SERVES 4 TO 6

PREP TIME: 10 minutes • **COOK TIME:** 4 hours

GI (Diarrhea), Nausea, Swallowing (includes mouth and throat soreness)

Chicken thighs are inexpensive and ideal for the slow cooker because it's almost impossible to overcook them. From the long, slow cook emerges a rich delicious sauce, with the miso providing a salty sweetness. Miso is an umami taste that's often tolerated more than other flavors. Serve over a bed of brown rice and sautéed bok choy, or white rice if you can't easily digest the brown rice. Bok choy is a surprisingly good source of calcium.

¼ cup white miso

2 tablespoons coconut oil, melted

2 tablespoons honey

1 tablespoon unseasoned
   rice wine vinegar

2 garlic cloves, thinly sliced

1 teaspoon minced fresh ginger root

1 cup chicken broth

8 boneless, skinless chicken thighs

2 scallions, white and
   green parts, sliced

1 tablespoon sesame seeds

1. In a slow cooker, combine the miso, coconut oil, honey, vinegar, garlic, and ginger root, mixing well. Add the broth and the chicken, and toss to combine. Cover and cook on high for 4 hours.

2. Transfer the chicken and sauce to a serving dish. Garnish with the scallions and sesame seeds, and serve. Store leftovers in the refrigerator for up to a week.

SUBSTITUTION: You can use chicken drumsticks instead of thighs, an equally tasty and economical alternative.

PER SERVING (4 PORTIONS): Calories: 320; Total fat: 15g; Sodium: 1,020mg; Carbohydrates: 17g; Fiber: 1g; Protein: 32g;

Dill Salmon with Cucumber-Radish Salad

SERVES 4

PREP AND COOLING TIME: 10 minutes and • **COOK TIME:** 20 minutes

Nausea, Taste Changes, Weight Loss

Oven-poached salmon is the star of this light salad. If you want to avoid food smells, stay out of the kitchen while it's cooking, and eat this delightful dish cold.

1 tablespoon extra-virgin olive
   oil, plus more for brushing
4 (3- to 4-ounce) salmon fillets
2 to 3 dill sprigs (keep the fronds)
1 shallot, sliced
½ cup dry white wine
2 teaspoons kosher salt, divided
¼ teaspoon freshly ground
   black pepper

2 cups sliced escarole
8 radishes, quartered
1 English cucumber, seeded
   and chopped
2 teaspoons minced dill fronds
1 tablespoon fresh lemon juice
Lemon slices, for garnish

1. Preheat the oven to 375°F. Brush a 9-inch square baking dish with olive oil. Place the salmon fillets, skin-side down, in the dish. Scatter the dill sprigs and shallot over the fish, then add the wine, 1 teaspoon of salt, and the pepper. Cover with aluminum foil, and bake until the fish is firm, 20 to 25 minutes.

2. Transfer the salmon fillets to a plate, and let them cool completely. Discard the remaining contents of the pan.

3. While the fish is cooling, in a medium bowl, combine the escarole, radishes, cucumber, and dill. Add the lemon juice, 1 tablespoon of olive oil, and the remaining teaspoon of salt. Toss well. Mound the salad on four plates, top with the salmon, garnish with the lemon slices, and serve.

PER SERVING: Calories: 361; Total fat: 23g; Sodium: 3,177mg;
Carbohydrates: 5g; Fiber: 1g; Protein: 27g

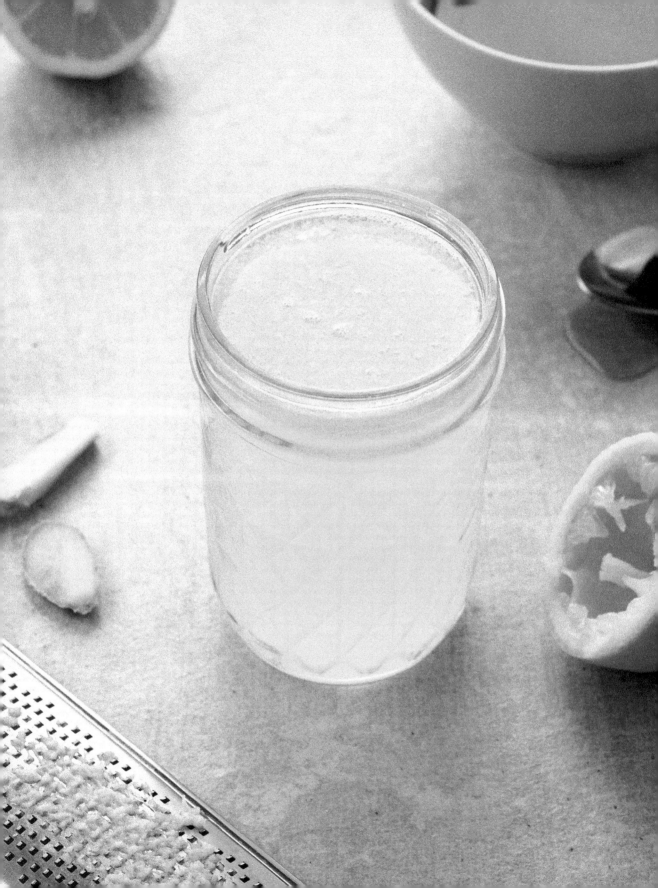

9

Drinks and Tonics

Spinach Ginger Smoothie

SERVES 2

PREP TIME: 10 minutes

GI (diarrhea and constipation), Nausea,
Swallowing (includes mouth and throat soreness)

Fresh ginger works alongside medications to soothe nausea. Ginger is also an effective antimicrobial and anti-inflammatory spice that calms digestive difficulties. It's best during treatment to use fresh ginger, but not more than a tablespoon daily. If you're sensitive to food smells, here's a valuable technique to use when drinking. Cover the smoothie with a lid and drink through a paper or plastic straw.

2 cups unsweetened plain soy milk

2 tablespoons ground flaxseed

5 cups fresh, or 2½ cups
   frozen, spinach leaves

1 frozen banana

1 ripe pear, chopped

2 tablespoons (2 inches)
   grated fresh ginger root

In the bowl of a blender, combine the milk, flaxseed, spinach leaves, banana, pear, and ginger root. Blend on high for 30 seconds, then pulse for 1 to 2 minutes until liquefied, and serve.

SUBSTITUTION: Replace the pear with a chopped, unpeeled apple for the additional pectin. Both the pectin and the banana can help firm stools. For additional calories, use whole milk or full-fat coconut milk instead of soy milk.

PER SERVING (1 CUP): Calories: 243; Total fat: 8g; Sodium: 149mg; Carbohydrates: 37g; Fiber: 9g; Protein: 12g

Turmeric Healing Smoothie

SERVES 2

PREP TIME: 5 minutes

Nausea, Taste Changes

Smoothies are a tasty way to pack more nutrition into your day as you are fighting nausea and dry mouth. This smoothie offers the tropical flavors of refreshing pineapple, mango, and coconut, along with the anti-inflammatory benefits of turmeric, which may be especially helpful for head and neck radiation side effects. Studies show the active ingredient in turmeric, curcumin, may slow the progression of head and neck tumors when combined with immunotherapy drugs. During treatment, because of its high antioxidant content, turmeric is recommended in food form only.

1 banana (fresh or frozen)
1 cup frozen pineapple chunks
1 cup frozen mango chunks
½ teaspoon turmeric

½ cup coconut milk (the type in the carton), or dairy milk
½ cup water

In a blender bowl, combine the banana, pineapple, mango, turmeric, milk, and water. Blend until it reaches your desired consistency, and serve.

MAKE IT EVEN EASIER: Buy fruit that is already precut and frozen. A frozen banana makes this milkshake creamier, so freeze ripened bananas.

PER SERVING (1 CUP): Calories: 183; Total fat: 3g; Sodium: 29mg; Carbohydrates: 40g; Fiber: 4g; Protein: 4g

5 INGREDIENTS OR FEWER · 30 MINUTES OR LESS · ONE-POT

Cranberry Grape Smoothie

SERVES 2
PREP TIME: 5 minutes

GI (constipation), Swallowing (includes mouth
and throat soreness), Taste Changes

Grapes have a compound, resveratrol, that we usually only associate with wine and heart health. In this recipe, you can drink your resveratrol without the alcohol and still reap the benefits of lowered inflammation and lung health. Studies show it may also slow cancer growth. Most of the benefits are found in the grape skins. This smoothie offers the right amount of tartness from cranberry juice, a good choice for when metallic and bitter tastes take over.

1 cup 100% cranberry
  juice, divided
2 teaspoons chia seeds, divided
1 cup red seedless grapes, divided

1 cup frozen organic
  strawberries, divided
½ cup unsweetened
  almond milk, divided

In the bowl of a blender, combine ½ cup of cranberry juice, 1 teaspoon of chia seeds, ½ cup of grapes, ½ cup of strawberries, and ¼ cup of milk and blend for 1 minute. Add the other half of all of the ingredients, and blend for 1 to 2 minutes, then serve.

SUBSTITUTION: Feel free to use a different frozen fruit combination—for example, for mouth sores, try replacing the cranberry juice with apple juice, and replacing the strawberries with a non-citrus fruit such as pears. If you have a dry mouth, tart foods such as cranberry juice can stimulate saliva to moisten and dry it. When food is flavorless, freeze the grapes first.

PER SERVING (1 CUP): Calories: 190; Total fat: 3g; Sodium: 30mg; Carbohydrates: 44g; Fiber: 5g; Protein: 3g

Pomegranate Mint Lemonade

SERVES 2

PREP AND STEEPING TIME: 5 minutes and 2 hours

Nausea, Swallowing (includes mouth and throat soreness), Taste Changes

It's disappointing when some foods just taste off. To remedy this, try tart drinks such as lemonade. This lemonade has added nutrients from pomegranate juice and herbal mint. Fresh mint contains an antispasmodic ingredient, can help with digestion, and is rich in antioxidants. Laboratory studies show it may even reduce the toxic effects of radiation. If your appetite is affected, make sure to drink this before or after meals rather than during. Drinking with meals will fill you up before you eat enough.

1 cup 100% pomegranate juice
½ cup lemon juice
Maple syrup

½ cup sparkling mineral
   water or water
¼ cup mint leaves

In a pitcher, combine the pomegranate juice, lemon juice, and maple syrup to taste. Mix well. Add the sparkling water. Top with the mint leaves, cover, and let steep in the refrigerator for 2 hours. Serve over ice.

MAKE IT EVEN EASIER: Mint is incredibly easy to grow. Buy a pot and keep it near your kitchen window. Chop a few leaves when you need to soothe digestion, add an anti-inflammatory herb, or flavor salads, grains, and drinks. A spearmint known as Nana mint has a softer and cooling flavor.

PER SERVING (1 CUP): Calories: 89; Total fat: 1g; Sodium: 20mg; Carbohydrates: 23g; Fiber: 0g; Protein: 0g

Turmeric Golden Milk Tea

SERVES 5

PREP AND STEEPING TIME: 10 minutes and 5 minutes • **COOK TIME:** 5 minutes

GI (diarrhea), Nausea, Swallowing (includes mouth and throat soreness)

Sometimes, between meals, you want a warm, comforting, and slightly sweet snack that's also healthy and anti-inflammatory. Snacks should provide your body with a balance of protein, carbohydrates, and fat for sustained energy. Next time you find yourself craving something warm, savory, and sweet, whip up a simple mug of this to sip on.

2 cups boiling water
3 bags ginger tea
3 cups unsweetened oat
  milk, warmed

1 teaspoon ground cinnamon
1½ teaspoons ground turmeric
1 teaspoon ground ginger
2 teaspoons maple syrup

1. In a large glass measuring cup or medium bowl, pour the boiling water over the tea bags. Steep for 5 minutes. Remove the tea bags, and add the oat milk, cinnamon, turmeric, ginger, and maple syrup.

2. Transfer the mixture to a blender, and blend until frothy, about 20 seconds. Divide into 5 mugs and serve warm.

PREP AHEAD: To make ahead, cool the tea and then store in the refrigerator for up to 1 week or portion into individual 1-cup servings and freeze for up to 2 months. To serve, reheat refrigerated or frozen golden milk in the microwave or on the stovetop. Sprinkle the hot milk tea with more cinnamon, if desired.

SUBSTITUTION: For a milder flavor, reduce the cinnamon and ginger. Try using other types of unsweetened nondairy milk, such as soy, rice, almond, cashew, or coconut; keep in mind that only soy milk has the protein to match dairy milk.

PER SERVING: Calories: 91; Total fat: 3g; Sodium: 87mg;
Carbohydrates: 13g; Fiber: 1g; Protein: 5g

Lemon and Ginger Tonic

SERVES 1

PREP AND CHILL TIME: 10 minutes and overnight

GI (diarrhea), Nausea, Swallowing (includes mouth and throat soreness)

This tonic is a mixture of lemon, ginger, and maple syrup. In addition to its numerous applications in beverages, you can use it to marinate chicken or shrimp. If you love the taste of lemon and have a dry mouth, feel free to squeeze a bit more into this recipe.

1 cup water

¼ cup freshly squeezed lemon juice

2 tablespoons maple syrup

2 teaspoons grated fresh ginger root

1. In an airtight jar, combine the water, lemon juice, maple syrup, and ginger root, and shake until the maple syrup is dissolved. Refrigerate for 24 hours before using so the ginger can permeate the mixture.

2. To make a beverage, pour 2 tablespoons of the tonic into a tall glass filled with ice. Add cold green tea, sparkling water, or seltzer, and serve.

PREP AHEAD: Make this ahead of time, because it stores in the refrigerator for up to a week.

PER SERVING (2 TABLESPOONS): Calories: 16;
Total fat: 0g; Sodium: 0mg; Carbohydrates: 4g; Fiber: 0g; Protein: 0g

Carrot Tomato Beet Juice

SERVES 2

PREP TIME: 5 minutes

Anemia, Fatigue, Taste Changes

Beets are a valuable addition when you need to increase your iron intake. In this juice, the beets, together with carrots, provide sweetness and an earthy taste. The tomatoes provide an umami flavor balance for sweetness. This combination also covers up bitter or too-salty tastes. Keep the beet greens for another cooked dish; they are among the most mineral-rich foods you can find.

2 medium beets, peeled,
  cooked and chopped (or
  2 canned beets, chopped)
2 medium tomatoes, diced

2 medium carrots, chopped
1 tablespoon lemon juice, to taste
1 cup water

If you own a juicer: Juice the beets, tomatoes, and carrots together. Then add the lemon juice and water to taste.

If you do not own a juicer: In a blender bowl, combine the water, beets, tomatoes, carrots, and lemon juice, and blend on high for 2 to 3 minutes. Strain the juice into a bowl. Add more water, if required, to get the right consistency.

SUBSTITUTION: Feel free to add other produce. For a sweeter juice, use 2 medium apples, or use pomegranate juice instead of tomatoes. Sweeter foods are usually better tolerated when food loses flavor or taste strange. For a spicy kick that aids digestion, you can add 1 to 2 inches of fresh ginger root, too.

PER SERVING (1 CUP): Calories: 84; Total fat: 1g; Sodium: 112mg; Carbohydrates: 19g; Fiber: 6g; Protein: 3g

Warm Vegetable Smoothie

SERVES 4

PREP TIME: 5 minutes • **COOK TIME:** 3 minutes

GI (constipation), Swallowing, Weight Loss

Many patients want colder foods for side effects, such as nausea and sensitivity to cooking smells, but sometimes you just need something warm. This warm vegetable smoothie packs in nutrition and protein with balanced flavors. The concept was developed by a dietitian who called them "smoupies," to help patients gain nutrition and maintain weight during treatments and after surgeries. Because all the ingredients are already cooked and soft, you can just place everything in a blender and whir for a savory smoothie.

2 cups soy milk, divided

1 cup cooked carrots

¼ cup cooked butternut squash

½ cup pureed canned white beans

½ teaspoon turmeric

2 scoops protein powder of choice

1. In the bowl of a blender, combine 1 cup of the soy milk, carrots, squash, beans, and turmeric, and blend. Add the other cup of soy milk, and blend it together on high for 2 to 3 minutes.

2. Remove from the blender. In a saucepan, heat the mixture gently over low heat, and whisk in protein powder slowly until mixed thoroughly, about 3 minutes. Serve warm.

MAKE IT EVEN EASIER: To cook carrots, the easiest method is to put them in a saucepan and cover with water. Bring to a boil, then simmer about 20 minutes. Keep the cooking liquid for the smoothie, and then you can make it as thick or thin as you need.

PER SERVING (1 CUP): Calories: 143; Total fat: 2g; Sodium: 120mg; Carbohydrates: 16g; Fiber: 4g; Protein: 14g

Strawberry Banana Smoothie

SERVES 2
PREP TIME: 5 minutes

Fatigue, Swallowing (includes mouth and throat soreness), Weight Loss

Protein shakes are often recommended for cancer patients. You can now find a protein shake for every need—from organic vegan drinks to shakes that help balance blood sugar. They taste much better when frozen and blended, resembling a milkshake. Smoothies can be sipped throughout the day for hydration and extra protein. Emerging data reveals a link between dairy and prostate cancer, so use nondairy milk and yogurt so that your smoothie is dairy-free but still nutritious. Omit the strawberries if you have mouth sores.

2 medium bananas

2 cups frozen strawberries

¾ cup plain 2% Greek yogurt

1 cup unsweetened almond milk

In the bowl of a blender, combine the bananas, strawberries, yogurt, and milk and blend until smooth. If you would like it thicker, use frozen banana chunks.

FLAVOR BOOST: Feel free to add a tablespoon of a sweetener of your choice for a sweeter smoothie; or, replace milk with a vegan protein shake, and coconut- or oat-based yogurt to make it lactose-free but still flavorful. The vegan shakes have as much protein as milk-based drinks, usually over 20 grams.

PER SERVING (1 CUP): Calories: 266; Total fat: 4g; Sodium: 93mg; Carbohydrates: 56g; Fiber: 8g; Protein: 6g

Blackberry Chia Cooler

SERVES 2
PREP TIME: 5 minutes

GI (diarrhea and constipation), Nausea, Swallowing
(includes mouth and throat soreness)

A fruit cooler is an alternative to a heavy milkshake, and hits all the hydration notes. This drink is not too sweet, but you can always add maple syrup to sweeten as needed. Chia and blackberries are a natural way to help move bowels, especially after taking pain medication. Chia seeds also contain omega-3 fatty acids, which help maintain weight during cancer treatment. You can make this recipe into ice pops to combat nausea. Omit the lemon if you're advised to stay away from acidity for mouth sores or soreness.

2 cups frozen blackberries
2 tablespoons chia seeds
¼ cup freshly squeezed lemon juice
2 cups club soda

½ cup crushed ice, divided
 into two glasses
Basil leaves for garnish, optional

In the bowl of a blender, combine the blackberries, chia seeds, lemon juice, and club soda, and blend for 3 minutes. Let it sit a few minutes, and blend again so the drink does not become clumpy. Pour the drink over ice. Serve with basil leaves for garnish (if using).

FLAVOR BOOST: Feel free to add fresh basil or some fresh ginger into the cooler while it's blending if you want a sharper flavor. If you want it lighter, add ½ cup more club soda to each drink.

PER SERVING (1 CUP): Calories: 201; Total fat: 9g; Sodium: 8mg;
Carbohydrates: 26g; Fiber: 17g; Protein: 7g

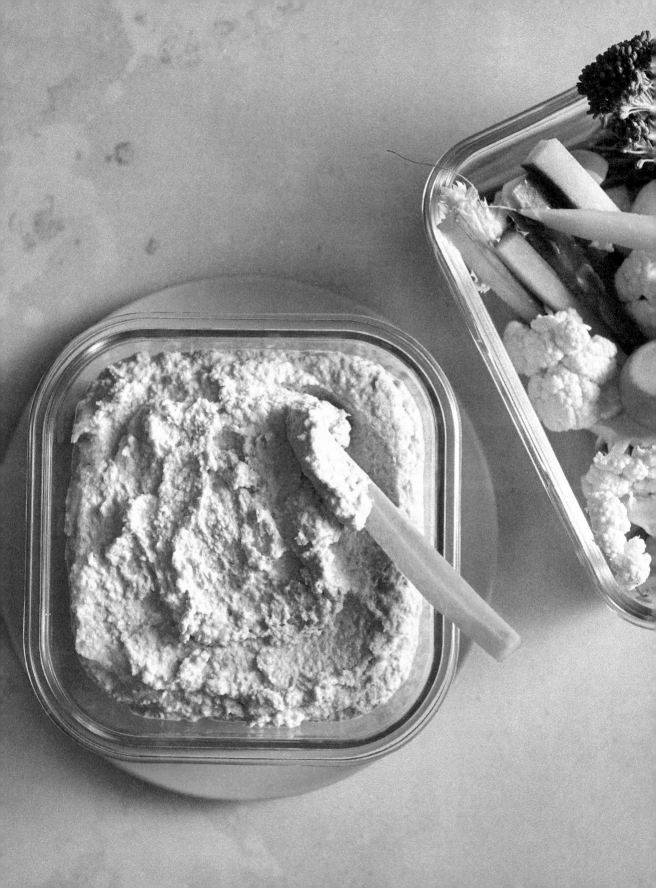

10

Staples and Condiments

Chicken Bone Broth

MAKES 6 SERVINGS

PREP TIME: 15 minutes, plus overnight to chill • **COOK TIME:** 18 hours

GI (diarrhea), Nausea, Swallowing (includes mouth and throat soreness)

This broth offers nourishment when appetite wanes and GI difficulties emerge. You can choose to make this broth with chicken bones (very budget-friendly) or vegetarian, with savory mushrooms (see Substitution). You can't get around the cooking time, because it takes a long time for the heady flavor to emerge. Freeze leftover broth in large-portioned ice cube trays with a cover for up to three months.

6 quarts water

2 pounds chicken bones

4 large carrots, chopped

8 celery stalks, chopped

1 large white onion, halved

1 garlic bulb, top removed

1 tablespoon sea salt

1 tablespoon black peppercorns

2 to 3 teaspoons dried thyme

¼ cup chopped fresh parsley, optional

1. In a slow cooker, combine the water, chicken bones, carrots, celery, onion, garlic, salt, peppercorns, and thyme. Turn the heat to medium-high, heat until nearly boiling, then reduce to simmer for 18 to 24 hours.

2. When 30 minutes remain, add the parsley.

3. Remove from the heat, and let it cool overnight in the refrigerator. In the morning, remove any congealed fat from the top of the bowl, strain out the vegetables and bones, and discard them. Enjoy the broth warm, and store the remaining broth in the refrigerator for up to 4 days or in the freezer for up to 3 months.

SUBSTITUTION: Make a nourishing vegetarian mushroom broth without the chicken bones. Sauté 2 pounds of sliced mushrooms, and substitute vegetable broth for the water. Add the rest of the ingredients, and cook as directed, for at least 2 hours. This broth will be more flavorful the longer you cook it.

PER SERVING (1 CUP): Calories: 25; Total fat: 0g; Sodium: 900mg; Carbohydrates: 2g; Fiber: 0g; Protein: 3g

Vegetable Broth

SERVES 8

PREP AND COOLING TIME: 10 minutes and 20 minutes • **COOK TIME:** 3 to 4 hours

GI (diarrhea), Nausea, Swallowing (includes mouth and throat soreness)

Sip this broth as is, or dip bread in to make it easier to chew. You can use this stock for any vegetable soup, grain, or rice dish. The minerals in the soup stay intact no matter how long you cook it, so broth is a valuable addition to your meals. Add rice to make this dish more filling. If you're concerned about arsenic in rice, measure one part rice to six parts water. Cook the rice until tender, and then drain and rinse before serving.

1 yellow onion, halved

1 garlic bulb, top cut off

4 carrots, coarsely chopped

4 celery stalks, coarsely chopped

1 ginger knob, coarsely chopped

1 gallon water

2 teaspoons dried thyme

1 tablespoon whole peppercorns

1 tablespoon kosher salt

1. In a large pot, combine the onion, garlic, carrots, celery, and ginger. Add the water, and turn the heat to medium-high. Bring the broth to a boil, then reduce the heat to a low simmer, add the thyme, peppercorns, and salt, cover, and cook 3 to 4 hours.

2. Let it cool for 20 minutes, and then, using a mesh strainer, strain the broth and toss (or reuse) the leftover vegetables. Serve immediately. Whatever broth you don't use, allow to cool to room temperature for no more than 2 hours before storing it in the refrigerator for up to 5 days or in the freezer for up to 3 months.

SUBSTITUTION: Feel free to add different herbs, such as fresh parsley or a bay leaf. For less salt, use a salt-free blend. Add sour cream for a heartier soup and additional calcium, but omit for nausea and diarrhea.

PER SERVING (1 CUP): Calories: 10; Total fat: 0g; Sodium: 900mg; Carbohydrates: 3g; Fiber: 0g; Protein: 0g

Olive Tapenade

SERVES 8 TO 9
PREP TIME: 10 minutes

Swallowing (includes mouth and throat soreness), Taste Changes, Weight Loss

Sometimes treatments can make foods taste overly sweet. If that's the case, turn to vegetables and tapenades for flavor enhancers and small snacks. A tapenade boosts the calories in small bites when weight loss is an issue. This tapenade can go well on the Everything Bagel–Seasoned Almond Flour Crackers (page 51), or on top of a protein of your choice. Also, choose cold, crisp vegetables such as celery, carrots, or radishes to dip. This tapenade has quite a bit of salt, so eat in small portions.

2 cups pitted kalamata olives
3 tablespoons capers, drained
1 garlic clove, minced
2 tablespoons chopped fresh parsley

2 tablespoons chopped fresh thyme
Juice of ½ lemon
¼ cup extra-virgin olive oil
Freshly ground black pepper, optional

In a food processor, combine the olives, capers, garlic, parsley, and thyme, and pulse 10 to 15 times. Add the lemon juice and olive oil. Pulse 5 to 10 more times, or until it reaches the desired consistency. Add black pepper to taste (if using) or more lemon juice, if desired.

FLAVOR BOOST: Feel free to add other herbs, such as fresh basil or oregano, or your own unique blend to mask flavors. You can also use other olive varieties or a mix of different pitted olives if you'd like.

PER SERVING (2 TABLESPOONS): Calories: 101; Total fat: 10g; Sodium: 323mg; Carbohydrates: 3g; Fiber: 1g; Protein: 0g

DIY Marinara Sauce

SERVES 8

PREP TIME: 5 minutes · **COOK TIME:** 1 hour

Swallowing (not mouth and throat soreness), Taste Changes

At times, foods may lose all flavor. Bring in different textures with sauces to top different types of foods. The umami flavors, here in tomatoes, are usually well-tolerated, except in cases of acid reflux. This sauce can be frozen for up to three months. Defrost and use it to top Edamame Spaghetti with Turkey Meatballs (page 100).

1 tablespoon extra-virgin olive oil

2 tablespoons diced garlic

1 medium yellow onion, diced

2 teaspoons dried oregano

1 teaspoon cayenne pepper

2 tablespoons red wine vinegar

2 (28-ounce) cans crushed tomatoes

Kosher salt

Freshly ground black pepper

¼ cup white sugar

1. In a 2-quart saucepan, heat the olive oil over medium heat, and add the garlic. Sauté the garlic for 1 minute. Add the onion, and sauté for another minute. Then add the oregano, cayenne pepper, red wine vinegar, crushed tomatoes, and salt and pepper to taste.

2. Reduce the heat to low, cover the pan, and let it simmer for 30 to 45 minutes, stirring every so often. After 45 minutes, use a whisk to break the sauce down a bit more, depending on the consistency you desire.

3. Add the sugar (it makes the sauce less acidic), and let it simmer for 15 more minutes. Add more salt, black pepper and even more sugar to taste, if necessary. Serve warm or store for later use.

FLAVOR BOOST: Add extra herbs, such as fresh basil, or vegetables, such as zucchini or carrots, to add more nutrients.

PER SERVING (½ CUP): Calories: 82; Total fat: 2g; Sodium: 249mg; Carbohydrates: 15g; Fiber: 4g; Protein: 2g

Garlic-Herb Marinated Tempeh or Tofu

SERVES 3

PREP TIME: 10 minutes, plus 20 minutes to marinate • **COOK TIME:** 20 minutes

Anemia, Fatigue, Taste Changes

Tempeh and tofu have very subtle flavors on their own, but they can be dressed up easily. Marinating these plant-based proteins in savory broth, tangy vinegar, and anti-inflammatory herbs and spices makes a wonderful base for many dishes.

8 ounces tempeh, or 14 ounces tofu
2 tablespoons olive oil
¼ cup vegetable broth or water
1 tablespoon white wine vinegar
3 garlic cloves, minced

1½ teaspoons dried thyme
½ teaspoon salt
½ teaspoon freshly ground
   black pepper

1. Preheat the oven to 400°F. Line a sheet pan with parchment paper.

2. If using tempeh, slice it crosswise into 1-inch-thick slices. If using tofu, press the tops and sides gently with a paper towel to remove extra water. Halve it lengthwise and press the slices again with a paper towel. Cut the tofu into 1-inch cubes.

3. To make the marinade, in a large bowl combine the oil, broth, vinegar, garlic, thyme, salt, and pepper. Place the tempeh or tofu in the marinade and use a spoon to coat thoroughly. Let it marinate for at least 10 minutes, then flip or toss and marinate for 10 minutes more.

4. Pour the tofu or tempeh onto the sheet pan in a single layer. Pour any additional marinade onto the pan and bake for 15 to 20 minutes, until the tempeh or tofu is slightly browned.

REUSE TIP: Tempeh and tofu are the perfect proteins for so many recipes. Make a batch—or even a double batch—of this each week and add it to salad or wrap recipes from this book. Store in a storage container in the refrigerator for up to 6 days.

PER SERVING: Calories: 233; Total fat: 17g; Sodium: 298mg; Carbohydrates: 9g; Fiber: 0g; Protein: 14g

5 INGREDIENTS OR FEWER • ONE-POT

White Bean Dip

SERVES 4

PREP AND RESTING TIME: 5 minutes and 15 minutes • **COOK TIME:** 20 minutes

Anemia, GI (constipation), Swallowing (includes mouth and throat soreness)

Soft beans provide a lot of nutrition during treatments. This flavorful dip is satisfying and provides a balanced snack with all the nutritious elements: protein, carbohydrates, and iron from beans; heart-healthy fat and nutrient absorption from olive oil; and flavonoids from parsley. What are flavonoids? Specific compounds of kaempferol and quercetin, found in parsley, are now seen as cancer protective and provide anti-inflammatory and antioxidant properties.

2 garlic cloves
1 (15-ounce) can cannellini
  beans, drained and rinsed
1 tablespoon extra-virgin olive
  oil, plus more for drizzling

Juice of ½ lemon
Kosher salt
Freshly ground black pepper
2 tablespoons chopped
  fresh parsley

1. Preheat the oven to 400°F.

2. Wrap the garlic cloves in foil, and place them on a small sheet pan. Roast until soft, about 20 minutes. Unwrap carefully, and allow the garlic to cool for 15 minutes. When cool, mince the cloves.

3. In a food processor, combine the beans, roasted garlic, olive oil, lemon juice, and salt and pepper to taste or put the ingredients in a bowl and blend with a hand blender. Process until smooth but not runny.

4. Top with a drizzle of olive oil, lemon juice, and the parsley.

FLAVOR BOOST: For a delicious flavor twist, add some salsa with the pureed beans. Choose your level of spice.

PER SERVING (¼ CUP): Calories: 126; Total fat: 4g; Sodium: 41mg; Carbohydrates: 18g; Fiber: 6g; Protein: 6g

Mango Tropical Dip

SERVES 4

PREP TIME: 10 minutes

Nausea, Swallowing (includes mouth and throat soreness), Taste Changes

This dip is cooling to the tongue, easy to eat when chewing is difficult, and provides a refreshing mini-meal after waking from an afternoon nap. Cold foods are more appealing when foods may have an off taste. This dish may be tolerable with mild nausea, and the tropical fruit might even whisk you away for a moment to the islands.

1 ripe avocado, peeled and pitted
1 mango, cubed
1 garlic clove, minced

Juice of ½ lemon
Pinch cayenne pepper, optional

In a medium bowl, mash the avocado until smooth. Add the mango, and mash again until smooth. Add the garlic, lemon juice, and cayenne (if using). Mix well, and serve with fresh, crisp, sliced vegetables, crackers, or as a topping for fish.

SUBSTITUTION: Don't have mango? Keep everything else the same but use a hand blender to whip the avocado. Whipped avocado is light and creamy, and may encourage you to eat more when your appetite is low.

PER SERVING (¼ CUP): Calories: 133; Total fat: 8g; Sodium: 5mg; Carbohydrates: 17g; Fiber: 5g; Protein: 2g

Edamame Hummus

SERVES 5

PREP TIME: 10 minutes · **COOK TIME:** 5 minutes

Anemia, GI (constipation), Weight Loss

Edamame hummus is the perfect way to boost protein and antioxidants in dip form. The tahini paste has added calcium, but if you're allergic to sesame, omit it. This hummus tastes great on whole-grain crackers, chips, and fresh veggies, such as carrots, bell peppers, cucumber, tomatoes, broccoli, cauliflower, or celery. This recipe uses frozen edamame, so you can make it even if you don't have fresh edamame on hand.

8 ounces frozen shelled edamame

¼ cup tahini

Juice of 1 large lemon

1 garlic clove, halved

¾ teaspoon kosher salt

½ teaspoon ground cumin

2 to 4 tablespoons water

3 tablespoons extra-virgin olive oil

1. Microwave the frozen edamame for 2 to 3 minutes, or per package instructions.

2. In the bowl of a food processor (see Substitution), combine the edamame, tahini, lemon juice, garlic, salt, cumin, and 2 tablespoons of water. Puree the mixture until it's smooth. If it needs more liquid, add up to 2 more tablespoons of water, 1 tablespoon at a time.

3. With the food processor running, slowly drizzle in the olive oil 1 tablespoon at a time, blending well to incorporate after each addition. Serve immediately, store in the refrigerator for up to 7 days or in the freezer for up to 3 months. If frozen, thaw a container of the hummus in the refrigerator overnight before serving.

SUBSTITUTION: A food processor is best for this recipe, so you can drizzle the olive oil in slowly while the motor is running. If you're using a blender, add 1 tablespoon of oil at a time and pulse 5 to 10 times to incorporate.

PER SERVING: Calories: 202; Total fat: 17g; Sodium: 180mg; Carbohydrates: 8g; Fiber: 4g; Protein: 7g

Lemony Mustard Dressing

MAKES ABOUT 1½ CUPS
PREP TIME: 10 minutes

Swallowing (includes mouth and throat soreness), Taste Changes, Weight Loss

Dry mouth and thicker saliva often make eating uncomfortable, and may lead to infections in the mouth. Lemon juice can increase the production of saliva and ease side effects. This recipe is a naturally delicious salad dressing or a sauce to put over steamed asparagus or broccoli. You can even try it as a marinade for poultry, tofu, or seafood.

1 cup extra-virgin olive oil
¼ cup freshly squeezed lemon juice (about 2 lemons)
1 tablespoon agave syrup
1 teaspoon Dijon mustard

1 shallot, sliced
1 teaspoon grated lemon zest
1 teaspoon kosher salt
¼ teaspoon pepper

In the bowl of a blender or food processor, combine the olive oil, lemon juice, agave syrup, mustard, shallot, lemon zest, salt, and pepper. Process until smooth. Use right away, or refrigerate in an airtight container for up to 5 days.

SUBSTITUTION: Don't have agave syrup? Substitute maple syrup instead.

PER SERVING (2 TABLESPOONS): Calories: 180; Total fat: 20g; Sodium: 220mg; Carbohydrates: 2g; Fiber: 0g; Protein: 0g

Tofu-Basil Sauce

MAKES ABOUT 2 CUPS
PREP TIME: 10 minutes

Anemia, Swallowing (includes mouth and throat soreness), Weight Loss

This is a high-protein spin on pesto, which can be used to give pasta and bean dishes a flavorful nutritional boost. When you're buying tofu, look for calcium-set tofu, for an extra dose of calcium. Aim for 2 to 3 servings a day of foods with calcium because cancer treatment can take a toll on the bones.

1 (12-ounce) package silken tofu
½ cup chopped fresh basil
2 garlic cloves, lightly crushed
½ cup almond butter

1 tablespoon fresh lemon juice
1 teaspoon kosher salt
¼ teaspoon freshly ground
   black pepper

In the bowl of a blender or food processor, combine the tofu, basil, garlic, almond butter, lemon juice, salt, and pepper. Process until smooth. If it's too thick, thin it with a bit of water. Serve, or refrigerate in an airtight container for up to 5 days.

SUBSTITUTION: If you're sensitive to nuts, you can substitute sunflower seed butter for the almond butter.

PER SERVING (¼ CUP): Calories: 120; Total fat: 10g; Sodium: 290mg; Carbohydrates: 5g; Fiber: 2g; Protein: 6g

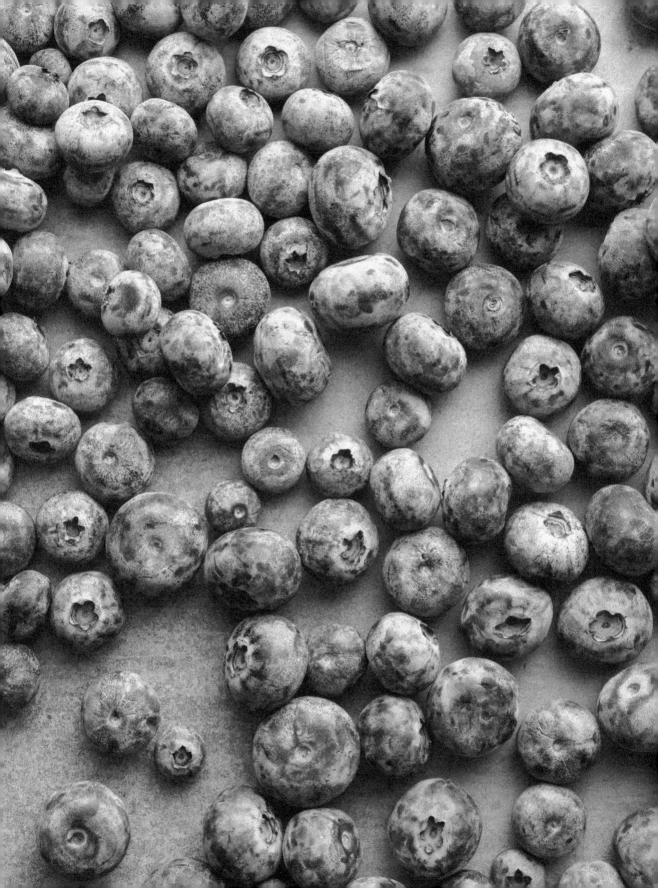

Measurement Conversions

VOLUME EQUIVALENTS	U.S. STANDARD	U.S. STANDARD (OUNCES)	METRIC (APPROXIMATE)
LIQUID	2 tablespoons	1 fl. oz.	30 mL
	¼ cup	2 fl. oz.	60 mL
	½ cup	4 fl. oz.	120 mL
	1 cup	8 fl. oz.	240 mL
	1½ cups	12 fl. oz.	355 mL
	2 cups or 1 pint	16 fl. oz.	475 mL
	4 cups or 1 quart	32 fl. oz.	1 L
	1 gallon	128 fl. oz.	4 L
DRY	⅛ teaspoon	—	0.5 mL
	¼ teaspoon	—	1 mL
	½ teaspoon	—	2 mL
	¾ teaspoon	—	4 mL
	1 teaspoon	—	5 mL
	1 tablespoon	—	15 mL
	¼ cup	—	59 mL
	⅓ cup	—	79 mL
	½ cup	—	118 mL
	⅔ cup	—	156 mL
	¾ cup	—	177 mL
	1 cup	—	235 mL
	2 cups or 1 pint	—	475 mL
	3 cups	—	700 mL
	4 cups or 1 quart	—	1 L
	½ gallon	—	2 L
	1 gallon	—	4 L

OVEN TEMPERATURES

FAHRENHEIT	CELSIUS (APPROXIMATE)
250°F	120°C
300°F	150°C
325°F	165°C
350°F	180°C
375°F	190°C
400°F	200°C
425°F	220°C
450°F	230°C

WEIGHT EQUIVALENTS

U.S. STANDARD	METRIC (APPROXIMATE)
½ ounce	15 g
1 ounce	30 g
2 ounces	60 g
4 ounces	115 g
8 ounces	225 g
12 ounces	340 g
16 ounces or 1 pound	455 g

Resources

GENERAL CANCER SUPPORT

Cancer Support Community (CancerSupportCommunity.org) has a chapter in every state.

Cancer.org

WeSpark.org

PatientPower.info/organization/mpn-research-foundation

Sharsheret.org

PowerfulPatients.org/whole-patient-support

CombatBootsNCancer.org

StupidCancer.org

CancerAdvocacy.org/resources/cancer-survival-toolbox

Finding accurate information:
Cancer.gov/about-cancer/managing-care/using-trusted-resources

EXERCISE

Silver Sneakers free exercise programs for Medicare

Survival2Strength.com

Joyn.co

NIA.NIH.gov/health/exercise-and-physical-activity-tracking-tools

Cancer.org/treatment/survivorship-during-and-after-treatment/
be-healthy-after-treatment/nutrition-and-physical-activity-during-an
d-after-cancer-treatment.html

RestorativeYogaTeachers.com

To find a certified cancer exercise trainer:
Certification2.ACSM.org/profinder?_ga=2.139239987.1600007473.1525799292
-1759941655.1523997371

ENVIRONMENT

EPA hotline (1-800-426-4791) for arsenic levels in your community. Community water systems are required by the EPA to publish an annual Consumer Confidence Report (CCR) on arsenic levels. Contact your water supplier or use the EPA's online tool to find your local CCR. EPA.gov/ccr

NIEHS.NIH.gov/health/materials/cancer_and_the_environment_508.pdf

INTEGRATIVE METHODS

Apps such as Calm, Insight Timer, website for Tara Brach (compassion) meditations.

Acupressure: MSKCC.org/cancer-care/patient-education/nausea-and-vomiting

SURVIVORSHIP

Cancer.net/survivorship/follow-care-after-cancer-treatment

Cancer.net/survivorship/healthy-living/healthy-living-after-cancer

NUTRITION FOR CANCER

AICR.org/cancer-prevention/food-facts

PearlPoint.org/nutrition

CancerDietitian.com

SurvivorStable.com

JeanLaMantia.com/jeans-nutrition-books/the-essential-cancer-treatment-nutrition
-guide-and-cookbook

CancerCare.org/tagged/nutrition

PCRM.org/good-nutrition/plant-based-diets

FDA.gov/media/102331/download

TASTE CHANGES

RebeccaKatz.com/blog/the-elephant-under-the-rug-transient-taste-changes-with
-cancer-therapy

RebeccaKatz.com/the-cancer-fighting-kitchen

SIDE EFFECTS

OralCancerFoundation.org/complications/mucositis

CancerResearchUK.org/about-cancer/coping/physically/diet-problems/managing

WCRF-UK.org/uk/here-help/eat-well-during-cancer/common-cancer-side-effects

https://www.OncologyNutrition.org/erfc

Cancer.gov/about-cancer/treatment/side-effects

LifeKitchen.co.uk/product/taste-flavour-digital-book

CookForYourLife.org/in-treatment

MSKCC.org/cancer-care/diagnosis-treatment/symptom-management/integrative
-medicine/herbs/search

ChemoCare.com/chemotherapy/side-effects/default.aspx

EatRight.org/health/diseases-and-conditions/cancer/chemotherapy-and-diet

Cancer.gov/publications/patient-education/eating-hints

HealthCare.Utah.edu/the-scope/shows.php?shows=0_d0sr337w

PODCASTS AND VIDEOS

SurvivorNet.com/?gclid=CjwKCAjw49qKBhAoEiwAHQVTo8ZPh3uX6kmyWOAY21 rxIBBiXL4GIfb55T3mxU7WyQ9_D7722ngquBoCVtEQAvD_BwE

Dana-Farber.org/health-library/articles/cancer-podcast-series/

CDC.gov/cancer/dcpc/resources/podcasts.htm

MyBreastMyHealth.com/podcasts/s2-ep26-is-there-such-a-thing-as-a-breast-cancer -diet-tamar-rothenberg: Dr. Tasha Gandamihardja is an Oncoplastic Breast Cancer and Reconstructive Surgeon.

InterludeCancerStories.com/interlude-podcast: Dr. Eleonora Teplinsky is a board-certified medical oncologist who also focuses on cancer risk-reduction and healthy living.

Research updates for all types of cancer. ASCOPost.com/podcasts/

References

Ambrosone, Christine B., Gary R. Zirpoli, Alan D. Hutson, William E. McCann, Susan E. McCann, William E. Barlow, Kara M. Kelly, et al. "Dietary Supplement Use During Chemotherapy and Survival Outcomes of Patients With Breast Cancer Enrolled in a Cooperative Group Clinical Trial (SWOG S0221)." *Journal of Clinical Oncology* 38, no. 8 (March 10, 2020): 804–814. ASCOPubs.org/doi/full/10.1200/JCO.19.01203.

American Cancer Society. "How to Tell a Child That a Parent Has Cancer." Accessed Nov. 10, 2021. Cancer.org/treatment/children-and-cancer/when-a-family-member-has-cancer/dealing-with-diagnosis/how-to-tell-children.html.

American Institute for Cancer Research. "Planning and Preparing." Accessed Nov. 10, 2021. AICR.org/cancer-survival/treatment-tips/during-treatment.

Andreyev, H. Jervoise N., Ann C. Muls, Clare Shaw, Richard R. Jackson, Caroline Gee, Susan Vyoral, and Andrew R. Davies. "Guide to Managing Persistent Upper Gastrointestinal Symptoms During and After Treatment for Cancer." *Frontline Gastroenterology* 8, no. 4 (Oct. 2017): 295–323. FG.BMJ.com/content/8/4/295.

Arun, P., A. Sagayaraj, S. M. Azeem Mohiyuddin, and D. Santosh. "Role of Turmeric Extract in Minimising Mucositis in Patients Receiving Radiotherapy for Head and Neck Squamous Cell Cancer: a Randomised, Placebo-Controlled Trial." *Journal of Laryngology & Otology* 134, no. 2 (2020): 159–64. DOI.org/10.1017/S0022215120000316.

ASCO 2019 Cancer Opinions Survey, The Harris Poll, September 2019. Accessed Nov. 10, 2021. ASCO.org/sites/new-www.asco.org/files/content-files/blog-release/pdf/2019-ASCO-Cancer-Opinion-Survey-Final-Report.pdf.

Bail, Jennifer R., Andrew D. Frugé, Mallory G. Cases, Jennifer F. De Los Santos, Julie L. Locher, Kerry P. Smith, Alan B. Cantor, Harvey J. Cohen, and Wendy Demark-Wahnefried. "A Home-Based Mentored Vegetable Gardening Intervention Demonstrates Feasibility and Improvements in Physical Activity and Performance

Among Breast Cancer Survivors." *Cancer* 124, no. 16 (Aug. 15, 2018): 3427–3435. DOI.org/10.1002/cncr.31559.

Berry, Leonard L., Tracey S. Danaher, Robert A. Chapman, and Rana L.A. Awdish. "Role of Kindness in Cancer Care." *Journal of Oncology Practice* 13, no. 11 (Nov. 1, 2017): 744–750. ASCOPubs.org/doi/10.1200/JOP.2017.026195.

Cancer.net. "Types of Cancer." Accessed Nov. 10, 2021, Cancer.net/cancer-types.

Cannioto, Rikki A., Alan Hutson, Shruti Dighe, William McCann, Susan E. McCann, Gary R. Zirpoli, William Barlow, et al. "Physical Activity Before, During, and After Chemotherapy for High-Risk Breast Cancer: Relationships With Survival." *Journal of the National Cancer Institute* 113, no. 1 (Jan. 2021): 54–63. DOI.org/10.1093/jnci/djaa046.

Childs, Caroline E., Philip C. Calder, and Elizabeth A. Miles 2019. "Diet and Immune Function." *Nutrients* 11, no. 8 (Aug. 16, 2019): 1933. DOI.org/10.3390/nu11081933.

Collins, Karen. "Nutrition Score Analysis Shows AICR Recommendations Significantly Lower Cancer Risk." American Institute for Cancer Research (blog). Accessed Nov. 10, 2021. AICR.org/resources/blog/nutrition-score-analysis-show s-aicr-recommendations -significantly-contribute-to-cancer-prevention.

Di Noia, Jennifer. "Defining Powerhouse Fruits and Vegetables: A Nutrient Den-sity Approach." *Preventing Chronic Disease* 11 (2014). DX.DOI.org/10.5888/pcd11.130390.

Eberle, Carolyn E., Dale P. Sandler, Kyla W. Taylor, and Alexandra J. White. "Hair Dye and Chemical Straightener Use and Breast Cancer Risk in A Large us Population of Black and White Women." *International Journal of Cancer* 147, no. 2 (July 15, 2020): 383–391. DOI.org/10.1002/ijc.32738.

Exercise Is Medicine. "Moving Through Cancer." Accessed Nov. 10, 2021. ExerciseIsMedicine.org/eim-in-action/moving-through-cancer.

Johnson, Skyler B., Matthew Parsons, Tanya Dorff, Meena S. Moran, John H. Ward, Stacey A. Cohen, Wallace Akerley, et al. "Cancer Misinformation and Harmful

Information on Facebook and Other Social Media: A Brief Report." *JNCI: Journal of the National Cancer Institute*, djab141 (July 22, 2021). DOI.org/10.1093/jnci/djab141.

Kaluza, Joanna, Holly R. Harris, Niclas Håkansson, and Alicja Wolk. "Adherence to The WCRF/AICR 2018 Recommendations for Cancer Prevention and Risk of Cancer: Prospective Cohort Studies Of Men And Women." *British Journal of Cancer* 122 (May 12, 2020): 1562–1570. DOI.org/10.1038/s41416-020-0806-x.

"Mind and Body Approaches for Cancer Symptoms and Treatment Side Effects: What the Science Says." *NCCIH Clinical Digest*, Oct. 2018. NCCIH.NIH.gov/health/providers
/digest/mind-and-body-approaches-for-cancer-symptoms-and-treatment-side
-effects-science.

National Cancer Institute. "Chemicals in Meat Cooked at High Temperatures and Cancer Risk." Accessed Nov. 10, 2021. Cancer.gov/about-cancer/causes-prevention
/risk/diet/cooked-meats-fact-sheet.

OncoLink. "Ginger: Health Benefits and Dietary Recommendations During Cancer Treatment." Reviewed Nov. 5, 2020. OncoLink.org/support/nutrition-and-cancer
/during-and-after-treatment/ginger-health-benefits-and-dietary-re
commendations-during-cancer-treatment.

Oncology Nutrition Dietetic Practice Group. *Oncology Nutrition for Clinical Practice*. 2nd ed. S.l.: American Dietetic Assn, 2021.

Ravasco, Paula, Isabel Monteiro-Grillo, and Maria Camilo. "Individualized Nutrition Intervention is of Major Benefit to Colorectal Cancer Patients: Long-Term Follow-Up of A Randomized Controlled Trial of Nutritional Therapy." *American Journal of Clinical Nutrition* 96, no. 6 (Dec. 2012): 1346–1353. DOI.org/10.3945/ajcn.111.018838.

Ravasco, Paula, Isabel Monteiro-Grillo, Pedro Marques Vidal, and Maria Ermelinda Camilo. "Dietary Counseling Improves Patient Outcomes: A Prospective, Randomized, Controlled Trial in Colorectal Cancer Patients Undergoing Radiotherapy." *Journal of Clinical Oncology* 23, no. 7 (March 01, 2005): 1431–1438. ASCOPubs.org/doi/10.1200
/JCO.2005.02.054.

Schroevers, Maya J., Vicki S. Helgeson, Robbert Sanderman, and Adelita V. Ranchor. "Type of Social Support Matters for Prediction of Posttraumatic Growth Among Cancer Survivors." *Psycho-Oncology* 19, no. 1 (Jan. 2010): 46–53. DOI.org/10.1002/pon.1501.

Sohn, Emily. "Simple Cooking Method Flushes Arsenic out of Rice." *Nature*, July 27, 2015. ScientificAmerican.com/article/simple-cooking-method-flushes-arsenic-out-of-rice.

Spencer, Christine N., Vancheswaran Gopalakrishnan, Jennifer McQuade, Miles C. Andrews, Beth Helmink, Md Abdul Wadud Khan, Elizabeth Sirmans, et al. "Abstract 2838: The Gut Microbiome (Gm) And Immunotherapy Response are Influenced by Host Lifestyle Factors." *Proceedings: AACR Annual Meeting* 70, no. 13 (July 2019): 2838. CancerRes.AACRJournals.org/content/79/13_Supplement/2838.

Tarpol, Jackie, and Vanessa Valero. *Nutrition During Cancer Treatment* (New York: New York-Presbyterian, 2015). NYP.org/documents/nutrition/nutrition-during-cancer-treatment-cookbook.pdf.

Trujillo, Elaine B., Katrina Claghorn, Suzanne W. Dixon, Emily B. Hill, Ashlea Braun, Elizabeth Lipinski, Mary E. Platek, Maxwell T. Vergo, and Colleen Spees. "Inadequate Nutrition Coverage in Outpatient Cancer Centers: Results of a National Survey." *Journal of Oncology* (2019): Article ID 7462940, 8 pages. DOI.org/10.1155/2019/7462940.

West, Malcolm A., Paul E. Wischmeyer, and Michael P. W. Grocott. "Prehabilitation and Nutritional Support to Improve Perioperative Outcomes." *Current Anesthesiology Reports* 7 (December 2017): 340–349. DOI.org/10.1007/s40140-017-0245-2.

Index

Acknowledgments

With much love and gratitude to my husband, and for my son. To my wise older sister, who never doubted I had a book in me. My family showed me by example true happiness is to help others, starting with my beloved grandfather, who walked uphill to read to hospital patients at the age of 90.

As Rabbi Hanina said, "I have learnt much from my teachers, more from my colleagues, and most from my students." To the cancer survivors in my practice who taught me about resilience, self-advocacy, and the struggle to be content with what you have—I applaud and thank you. To oncology dietitians, you are awesome professionals who did all the hard work before me.

To my mother and grandmother, who I never got to know because cancer took you away so very young, and to my aunt, who raised me. These astounding women created a blueprint of how to help others with challenges live to the fullest. This book is meant for all of you.

I couldn't have done this book without my recipe developer, Carrie Gabriel, MS, RD, founder of Steps 2 Nutrition. She's a talented chef and registered dietitian—an awesome combination. I deeply thank Callisto Media and their superb staff for making sure this book has accurate information for a vulnerable population.

About the Author

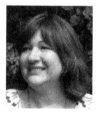 **TAMAR ROTHENBERG, MS, RDN,** is a registered dietitian nutritionist who specializes in nutrition for breast cancer thrivers in the private practice she founded, Nutrition Nom Nom, in Los Angeles. She has a certificate of training in vegetarian nutrition from the Academy of Nutrition and Dietetics, and is an adjunct professor of nutrition at Touro College, Los Angeles. She co-facilitated the study "Coping with Cancer in the Kitchen" at the Cancer Support Community of Los Angeles and published in *Nutrients*, October 2020.

Follow Tamar on her website, TamarRothenbergRD.com, and via Instagram @breastcancer.nutritionist, and join a community of fad-free nutrition for thrivers in a private Facebook group, A Fresh Start for Breast Cancer Thrivers.

Printed in the USA
CPSIA information can be obtained
at www.ICGtesting.com
CBHW072032250324
5818CB00005BA/15

9 781638 780373